Minimally Invasive Surgery in the Foot and Ankle

Editor

ANTHONY PERERA

FOOT AND ANKLE CLINICS

www.foot.theclinics.com

Consulting Editor
MARK S. MYERSON

September 2016 • Volume 21 • Number 3

ELSEVIER

1600 John F. Kennedy Boulevard • Suite 1800 • Philadelphia, Pennsylvania, 19103-2899

http://www.theclinics.com

FOOT AND ANKLE CLINICS Volume 21, Number 3
September 2016 ISSN 1083-7515, ISBN-13: 978-0-323-46256-3

Editor: Jennifer Flynn-Briggs
Developmental Editor: Meredith Clinton

Foot and Ankle Clinics (ISSN 1083-7515) is published quarterly by Elsevier, Inc., 360 Park Avenue South, New York, NY 10010-1710. Months of issue are March, June, September, and December. Periodicals postage paid at New York, NY, and additional mailing offices. Subscription price per year is $320.00 (US individuals), $466.00 (US institutions), $100.00 (US students), $360.00 (Canadian individuals), $560.00 (Canadian institutions), $215.00 (Canadian students), $460.00 (international individuals), $560.00 (international institutions), and $215.00 (international students). To receive student/resident rate, orders must be accompanied by name of affiliated institution, date of term, and the *signature* of program/residency coordinator on institution letterhead. Orders will be billed at individual rate until proof of status is received. Foreign air speed delivery is included in all *Clinics* subscription prices. All prices are subject to change without notice. **POSTMASTER:** Send address changes to *Foot and Ankle Clinics*, Elsevier Health Sciences Division, Subscription Customer Service, 3251 Riverport Lane, Maryland Heights, MO 63043. **Customer Service: 1-800-654-2452 (US and Canada). From outside of the United States and Canada, call 314-447-8871. Fax: 314-447-8029. E-mail: JournalsCustomerService-usa@ elsevier.com (for print support); JournalsOnlineSupport-usa@elsevier.com (for online support).**

Reprints. For copies of 100 or more, of articles in this publication, please contact the Commercial Reprints Department, Elsevier Inc., 360 Park Avenue South, New York, NY 10010-1710. Tel.: 212-633-3874; Fax: 212-633-3820; E-mail: reprints@elsevier.com.

Contributors

CONSULTING EDITOR

MARK S. MYERSON, MD
Medical Director, The Foot and Ankle Association, Inc., Baltimore, Maryland

EDITOR

ANTHONY PERERA, MBChB, MRCS, MFSEM, PG Dip(Med Law), FRCS (Orth)
Consultant Orthopaedic Foot and Ankle Surgeon, Spire Cardiff Hospital, BUPA Cromwell Hospital London and University Hospital of Wales, London, United Kingdom

AUTHORS

THOMAS BAUER, MD, PhD
Foot and Ankle Specialist, Department of Orthopedic Surgery, Ambroise Paré Hospital, West Paris University, Boulogne, France

GUILLAUME CORDIER, MD
Orthopaedic Surgeon, Orthopaedic Department, Mérignac Sport Clinic, Mérignac, France

MARTIN DI NALLO, MD
Fellow, Orthopaedic and Arthritis Specialist Centre, Sydney, New South Wales, Australia

STÉPHANE GUILLO, MD
Orthopaedic Surgeon, Orthopaedic Department, Mérignac Sport Clinic, Mérignac, France

GREGORY P. GUYTON, MD
Attending, Department of Orthopaedic Surgery, MedStar Union Memorial Hospital, Baltimore, Maryland

PETER LAM, MB BS (Hons), FRACS
Orthopaedic and Arthritis Specialist Centre, Sydney, New South Wales, Australia

MOSES LEE, MD
Department of Orthopedic Surgery, Yonsei Sarang Hospital, Seoul, Korea

SHU-YUAN LI, MD, PhD
Foot and Ankle Attending Surgeon, Foot and Ankle Center, Orthopaedic Department, Beijing Tongren Hospital, Capital Medical University, Beijing, China

FREDERICK MICHELS, MD
Orthopaedic Surgeon, Orthopaedic Department, AZ Groeninge Kortrijk, Kortrijk, Belgium

ROSLYN J. MILLER, FRCS (Tr&Orth)
Consultant Orthopaedic Foot and Ankle Surgeon, Department of Orthopaedics, Hairmyres Hospital, Lanarkshire, United Kingdom; Consultant Orthopaedic Foot and Ankle Surgeon, The London Orthopaedic Clinic, London, United Kingdom

STEPHEN PARSONS, FRCS (Tr&Orth)
Consultant in Trauma and Orthopaedics, Royal Cornwall Hospitals NHS Trust, Truro, United Kingdom

ANTHONY PERERA, MBChB, MRCS, MFSEM, PG Dip(Med Law), FRCS (Orth)
Consultant Orthopaedic Foot and Ankle Surgeon, Spire Cardiff Hospital, BUPA Cromwell Hospital London and University Hospital of Wales, London, United Kingdom

AISHA RAZIK, FRCS
Senior Specialist Registrar in Trauma and Orthopaedics, Foot and Ankle Unit, Epsom and St Helier University Hospitals NHS Trust, London, United Kingdom

DAVID J. REDFERN, FRCS (Tr&Orth)
Consultant Orthopaedic Surgeon, The London Foot and Ankle Centre, Hospital St John & St Elizabeth, St John's Wood, London, United Kingdom

A.H. SOTT, FRCS (Tr&Orth)
Consultant Orthopaedic Surgeon, Foot and Ankle Unit, Clinical Director, Trauma and Orthopaedics, Epsom and St Helier University Hospitals NHS Trust, London, United Kingdom

FILIP STOCKMANS, MD, PhD
Plastic Surgeon, Orthopaedic Department, AZ Groeninge Kortrijk; Department of Development and Regeneration, Faculty of Medicine, University of Leuven campus Kortrijk, Kortrijk, Belgium

TURAB ARSHAD SYED, MBBS, MRCS (GB), MFSEM (UK), DipSICOT, FRCS Eng (Tr&Orth), MSc (Bath)
Senior Fellow Foot and Ankle Surgery, Cardiff Regional Foot and Ankle Surgery Unit, Department of Trauma Orthopaedic Surgery, University Hospital Wales, Cardiff, United Kingdom

MICHAEL G. UGLOW, MBBS(Lond), FRCS (Tr&Orth)
Consultant Orthopaedic Surgeon, Department of Paediatric Orthopaedics, University Hospital Southampton, Southampton, United Kingdom

JOEL VERNOIS, MD
Sussex Orthopaedic Treatment Centre, Haywards Heath, United Kingdom; ICP, Paris, France

RICHARD WALTER, FRCS (Tr&Orth), MSc
Consultant in Trauma and Orthopaedics, Royal Cornwall Hospitals NHS Trust, Truro, United Kingdom

IAN WINSON, FRCS (Tr&Orth)
Consultant in Trauma and Orthopaedics, Sports and Orthopaedic Clinic, Bristol Spire Hospital, Bristol, United Kingdom

JERRY XING, MD
Fellow, Orthopaedic and Arthritis Specialist Centre, Sydney, New South Wales, Australia

JIAN-ZHONG ZHANG, MD
Professor; Foot and Ankle Attending Surgeon; Head, Foot and Ankle Center, Orthopaedic Department, Beijing Tongren Hospital, Capital Medical University, Beijing, China

YONG-TAO ZHANG, MS
Foot and Ankle Attending Surgeon, Orthopedics and Traumatology Department, Zibo Combinational Hospital of Chinese and Western Medicine, Zibo City, Shandong Province, China

Contents

of percutaneous surgery have not been promising. The authors have no experience of performing this osteotomy and report only on their management of the complications of this technique and their recommended treatment algorithm.

The traditional open surgical options for the treatment of metatarsalgia and lesser toe deformities are limited and often result in unintentional stiffness. The use of percutaneous techniques for the treatment of metatarsalgia and lesser toe deformities allows a more versatile and tailor-made approach to the individual deformities. As with all percutaneous techniques, it is vital that the surgeon engage in cadaveric training from surgeons experienced in these techniques before introducing them into his/her clinical practice.

Osteotomies of the calcaneus are powerful surgical tools, representing a critical component of the surgical reconstruction of pes planus and pes cavus deformity. Modern minimally invasive calcaneal osteotomies can be performed safely with a burr through a lateral incision. Although greater kerf is generated with the burr, the effect is modest, can be minimized, and is compatible with many fixation techniques. A hinged jig renders the procedure more reproducible and accessible.

First metatarsophalangeal joint arthrodesis plays a significant role in the management of symptomatic hallux rigidus/osteoarthritis of the 1st metatarsophalangeal joint. Several open and few percutaneous techniques have been described in the literature. This article describes and discusses a percutaneous technique that has been successfully used to achieve a pain-free stable and functional 1st metatarsophalangeal joint. All aspects of surgical indication and operative technique and details of patient-reported outcomes are presented with a referenced discussion.

The techniques for performing percutaneous osteotomies in treating deformities of the foot in children are presented along with a detailed description of the operative details. The author's use of minimal-access surgery for tibial, os calcis, and midfoot osteotomies is described using a cooled side-cutting burr that has not previously been described for use in the child's foot. The cancellous nature of the bones in the child are easily cut with the burr and the adjacent soft tissues are not damaged. The early experience of the healing times are not impaired and the complications associated with percutaneous scars seem to be negligible.

Roslyn J. Miller

Patients with peripheral neuropathy associated with ulceration are the
nemesis of the orthopedic foot and ankle surgeon. Diabetic foot syndrome
is the leading cause of peripheral neuropathy, and its prevalence continues
to increase at an alarming rate. Poor wound healing, nonunion, infection,
and risk of amputation contribute to the understandable caution toward
this patient group. Significant metalwork is required to hold these technically challenging deformities. Neuropathic Minimally Invasive Surgeries
is an addition to the toolbox of management of the diabetic foot. It may
potentially reduce the risk associated with large wounds and bony correction in this patient group.

Thomas Bauer

Hindfoot and midfoot fusions can be performed with percutaneous techniques. Preliminary results of these procedures are encouraging because
they provide similar results than those obtained with open techniques with
less morbidity and quick recovery. The best indications are probably fusions for mild-to-moderate reducible hindfoot and midfoot deformities in
fragile patients with general or local bad conditions. The main limit is linked
to the surgeon's experience in percutaneous foot surgery because a
learning curve with the specific tools is necessary before doing these
procedures.

Turab Arshad Syed and Anthony Perera

Haglund's syndrome encompasses several different pathologies,
including Haglund's deformity, insertional Achilles tendonopathy, retrocalcaneal bursitis, and superficial bursitis. Traditionally treated with open surgery, there is increasing interest in a more minimally invasive approach to
this difficult region to reduce complications and improve the rate and ease
of recovery. We review the evidence available for 2 of these techniques:
the endoscopic calcaneoplasty and percutaneous Zadek's calcaneal osteotomy (also known as Keck and Kelly's osteotomy). The senior author's
classification for management of the condition is presented as well as
describing his operative technique for these procedures.

Frederick Michels, Guillaume Cordier, Stéphane Guillo, Filip Stockmans, and
ESKKA-AFAS Ankle Instability Group

Chronic instability is a common complication of lateral ankle sprains. If
nonoperative treatment fails, a surgical repair or reconstruction may be
indicated. Today, endoscopic techniques to treat ankle instability are
becoming more popular. This article describes an endoscopic technique,
using a step-by-step approach, to reconstruct the ATFL and CFL with a

FOOT AND ANKLE CLINICS

Preface

Advances in Minimally Invasive Surgery of the Foot and Ankle— Percutaneous, Arthroscopic, and Endoscopic Operative Techniques

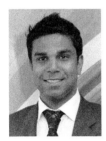

Anthony Perera, MBChB, MRCS,
MFSEM, PG Dip(Med Law), FRCS (Orth)
Editor

The development in our understanding of the foot and ankle over the last 20 years has given us a very good idea of what needs to be changed in order to correct most conditions. In addition, over the last 10 years, there has been a major focus on advances in implant technology and options to the extent that the reliability of achieving and maintaining that correction has also greatly improved. However, in contrast to other fields, for instance, trauma surgery where minimizing the approach is an important driver of change, little has changed with regard to the surgical approach in the foot and ankle.

Consider hallux valgus surgery for instance, where we have seen the approach actually increase. Compared with the Mitchell's and Wilson's osteotomies of yesteryear, it is now common to see a larger approach with a scarf or Ludloff osteotomy plus an open lateral release and an Akins' osteotomy. This is rightly so as these are better at achieving an appropriate correction and then holding this correction, but the end result is an operation that to a trauma surgeon is more like a grade II or III open fracture; it is unsurprising that stiffness, swelling, and soreness can be persistent bugbears that can hinder an excellent correction. Perhaps these complications do not get the recognition that they deserve because the literature relies on radiologic markers and outcomes scores that are not best suited to these issues; however, it is logical that minimizing the dissection, soft tissue, and periosteal injury should help to reduce these risks.

Attempts to develop minimally invasive surgery in the foot and ankle (arthroscopic ankle fusion and cheilectomy apart) have been met with some opposition, and rightly

Foot Ankle Clin N Am 21 (2016) xiii–xiv
http://dx.doi.org/10.1016/j.fcl.2016.06.001
1083-7515/16/© 2016 Published by Elsevier Inc.

so, as early techniques promoted the skin incision size over the importance of the basic principles of hallux valgus surgery and fixation as laid out by Barouk, Myerson, and others. We know that application of these principles is of fundamental importance and has enabled a disparate range of osteotomies to be successfully performed. Therefore, the challenge is to apply the same principles, but through a more minimally invasive, percutaneous, or arthroscopic/endoscopic approach.

This may require new technology to do existing procedures, modifying existing procedures or implants, or last, developing new procedures rather than just trying to do everything the same but through a smaller cut. This issue presents examples of each of these procedures that are being used for minimally invasive surgery around the world. It is very important to note that this is not intended as a surgical manual, and the only way to introduce these techniques in to your practice is to attend a cadaver course and learn hands on under the supervision of experts. The basic courses will commence with cheilectomy for hallux rigidus and Akins' osteotomy, and one should be very comfortable with the use of the instrumentation before embarking on the advanced courses to learn the more difficult techniques.

I would like to thank my mentor and friend, Dr Mark Myerson, for the opportunity to produce this issue and for everything that he has taught me.

Anthony Perera, MBChB, MRCS, MFSEM, PG Dip(Med Law), FRCS (Orth)
Spire Cardiff Hospital
Croescadarn Road
Cardiff, CF23 0XL, UK

E-mail address:
anthony@footandankleuk.com

Cheilectomy for Hallux Rigidus

Aisha Razik, FRCS, A.H. Sott, FRCS Tr&Orth*

KEYWORDS

- Hallux rigidus • Osteoarthritis first metatarsophalangeal joint • Cheilectomy
- Minimally invasive technique • Minimally invasive forefoot surgery • Arthrodesis
- Patient-reported outcomes

KEY POINTS

- Hallux rigidus (HR) is a clinical presentation associated with osteoarthritis of the first metatarsophalangeal joint.
- Impingement pain from osteophytes is worse at push-off and often progressive in nature.
- A cheilectomy is often an early part of surgical treatment of HR.
- Minimally invasive techniques have been increasingly used and the results postoperatively have been excellent.
- Time to recovery and patient satisfaction show promising results.

INTRODUCTION: NATURE OF THE PROBLEM

Hallux rigidus (HR) is a condition that is associated with degenerative changes affecting the first metatarsophalangeal joint.[1] It is associated commonly with osteoarthritis in the foot and is the second most common pathology affecting the great toe, after hallux valgus deformities. There has been some association with repetitive trauma, which can lead to posttraumatic arthritic changes, and commonly athletes, runners in particular, tend to present with symptoms of HR.

There is a female preponderance (2:1). Patients experience symptoms of pain, rubbing on shoes, and stiffness. Pain seems to be worse on push off gait and in dorsiflexion of the great toe. Pain is relieved with rest. As the disease progresses, the pain can become less severe as the range of movement is reduced.

Radiographs should be taken in the anteroposterior and lateral positions as weight bearing views. In the lateral views, dorsal osteophytes can be seen. There may be loss of joint space and evidence of bone cysts, subchondral sclerosis, widening or

The authors have nothing to disclose.
Trauma & Orthopaedics, Foot & Ankle Unit, Epsom & St Helier University Hospitals NHS Trust, Wrythe Lane, London SM5 1AA, UK
* Corresponding author.
E-mail address: Andrea.sott@esth.nhs.uk

flattening of the first metatarsal head and base of proximal phalanx and sesamoid hypertrophy (**Figs. 1** and **2**).

INDICATIONS AND CONTRAINDICATIONS

In the first instance, nonoperative treatment can be used to manage symptoms of HR in the form of nonsteroidal antiinflammatory medication, steroid injections, orthotics— stiff rigid insoles, rocker bottom shoes, shoe box stretching—and activity modifications (**Box 1**).

SURGICAL TECHNIQUE AND PROCEDURE
Preoperative Planning

- Systematic history and examination of patient.
- Standing weight bearing radiographic views of foot in anteroposterior and lateral positions.

Radiologic staging and clinical assessment would suggest that only grades 2 and 3 HR (osteophyte formation and some stiffness without midrange pain) should be addressed by dorsal cheilectomy. Certainly the best outcomes can be predicted in patients with isolated dorsal osteophytes and problems with rubbing on shoes but not displaying signs of midrange joint pain. We would, however, assess each patient on their merit, taking into account their history and physical findings, possibly placing less emphasis on the radiologic appearances when recommending minimally invasive cheilectomy. Based on our experience and our patients' satisfaction with this procedure, a patient may well benefit from cheilectomy even if adverse radiologic signs are present, as long as the consent process includes a frank discussion on the limitations and possible need for further surgery.

PREPARATION AND PATIENT POSITIONING

- This is a day case procedure, after which patients may be discharged on the same day of surgery.
- Consent for cheilectomy of the first metatarsophalangeal joint under intravenous sedation with or without general anesthesia is obtained.
- Patient is positioned supine, local protocol for sterile prepping is observed, extremity draping is performed, and no tourniquet is required (**Fig. 3**).

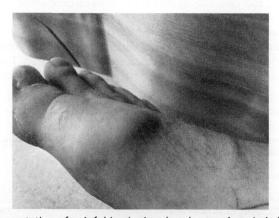

Fig. 1. Clinical presentation of painful impinging dorsal osteophyte in hallux rigidus.

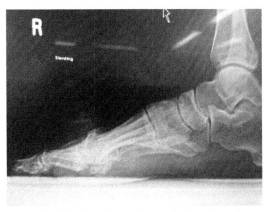

Fig. 2. Preoperative lateral weight-bearing radiograph showing advanced osteoarthritis of the first metatarsophalangeal joint with a large dorsal osteophyte.

- Ankle block is administered (20 mL bupivacaine 0.25%).
- Fluoroscopy available in the operating room.
- Optional arthroscopy equipment to check the joint postoperatively.

SURGICAL APPROACH

- Two skin incisions—1 dorsal medial portal and a second portal for the outflow cannula to allow lavage (**Fig. 4**).

SURGICAL PROCEDURE
Step One

Two keyhole incisions are used for 2-portal access. Dorsal incision 1.5 cm proximal and dorsal to the first metatarsophalangeal joint, developing the access with a periosteal elevator to create working space and the second portal, can be placed laterally for the cannula lavage of bony debris. The exact positioning of the working and lavage

---

Box 1
Indications/contraindications for minimally invasive cheilectomy for HR

Indications for surgical treatment of HR

1. Failure of nonsurgical treatment for painful osteophytes in HR

2. Impingement/dorsiflexion pain

Contraindications

1. Midrange pain without palpable osteophytes

2. Any sign of infection

Relative contraindications

3. Positive grind test

4. Predominantly plantar pain

5. Rest pain

Abbreviation: HR, hallux rigidus.

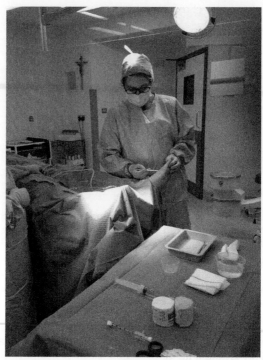

Fig. 3. Set up of the surgeon in operating theatre with patient positioning, available fluoroscopy applying local anesthesia block before minimally invasive cheilectomy.

portals are somewhat determined by the position and shape of the osteophyte, the surgeon's handedness, and other anatomic particulars of individual patients.

Step Two

A careful soft tissue pocket is created by using the minimally invasive periosteal elevator through the dorsal proximal portal so that access to the subperiosteum, osteophytes, and joint space arthritis is achieved. These osteophytes are removed with a handheld high-speed burr under radiographic guidance. The high-speed burr works via a torque and coolant system creating an accurate osteotomy/debridement with minimal thermal necrosis. The driver we use is designed specifically for foot

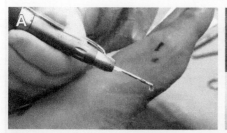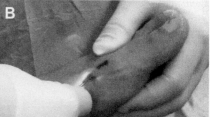

Fig. 4. (*A, B*) Access portal and water cooled burr to carry out removal of dorsal osteophyte in hallux rigidus.

surgery and has control of both speed and torque as well as having a built in saline feed onto the burr for cooling. These authors recommend that with the higher torque of this machine that 300 rpm is sufficient and, in using such a low speed, heat generation is minimal and so the risk of singe or burn to the skin also minimal. We have never experienced any skin burns in more than 300 cases performed.

As the bone is removed, it creates a fine paste, which is irrigated with normal saline via a cannula, which can further be extracted by digital pressure.

Step Three

Single-use instruments including a handheld curette/rasp can be used to smooth out any ridges with a final generous irrigation of the portals (**Figs. 5–7**).

Step Four

After careful and repeated lavage, portal sites are closed with SteriStrips. The forefoot is covered in protective bandaging (**Fig. 8**).

COMPLICATIONS AND MANAGEMENT

Swelling improves with time. The risk of infection increases with smoking and diabetes mellitus. Rare risks include scar sensitivity, nerve injury, and chronic regional pain syndrome. The risk of developing a deep vein thrombosis is less than 1% in minimally invasive cheilectomy and is reduced considerably by advising patients to be fully weight bearing immediately in an adapted postoperative shoe, using crutches if necessary.

POSTOPERATIVE CARE

The patient is advised to rest and elevate the leg in the immediate postoperative period. They can mobilize in a flat postoperative shoe and the dressings and bandaging can be removed after 5 to 7 days. Patients are most likely able to return to work within 1 to 2 weeks for sedentary jobs and 3 to 4 weeks for work requiring standing and walking. Patients can start driving usually 1 week after surgery in a comfortable but supportive rocker bottom trainer shoe.

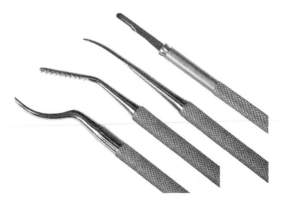

Fig. 5. Single-use instrument set (Wright medical Ltd) including a scalpel, 2 periosteal elevators and a rasp to facilitate access, creation of working cavity and removing bone debris after use of burr in minimally invasive surgery.

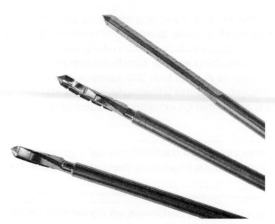

Fig. 6. A selection of 3.1-mm wedge burr (*top*) and 12-mm and 20-mm Shannon burrs (*middle, bottom*).

OUTCOMES

Outcomes of open dorsal cheilectomy for HR have shown promising results: 84% of patients experienced significant improvement in walking and 59% experienced improvement in pain using the MOXFQ when we assessed our cohort as part of an ongoing departmental audit (Sott AH, Ridgers S. Patient reported outcome after minimally invasive cheilectomy for HR at the Foot & Ankle unit Epsom & St Helier University Hospital NHS Trust Database. 2014 [unpublished data]). Minimally invasive dorsal cheilectomy has also shown excellent results. In our department, we looked at the possible difference in patient experience after cheilectomy depending on whether a percutaneous or open approach had been used. An independent assessor (research nurse) obtained MOXFQ and visual analog scale pain scores by telephoning a consenting cohort of patients at a minimum of 1 year postoperatively. This study of 47 patients, 22 of whom had minimally invasive cheilectomy and 25 open cheilectomy, showed significant improvement in pain scores using the MOXFQ pain scale (median preoperative score [35/64] and median postoperative score [7.5/64]).[2] These results are very reassuring and there are fewer reported incidences of infection and

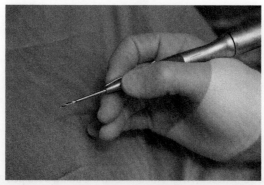

Fig. 7. Handheld 8-mm Shannon burr using a foot pedal to carry out high torque, low-speed water cooled cutting.

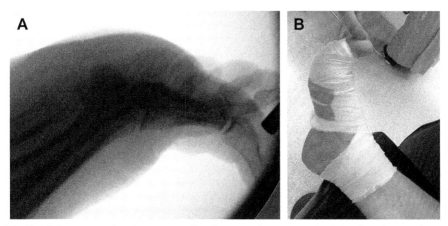

Fig. 8. (*A*) Intraoperative fluoroscopy showing complete removal of the dorsal osteophyte. (*B*) Clinical picture demonstrating the range of motion in a patient after cheilectomy.

postoperative complications in minimally invasive compared with open procedures. Patient satisfaction seems to be a positive indicator for the use of minimally invasive cheilectomy.

In our experience, the presence of plantar pain, rest pain, and a positive grind test certainly warrants a frank and open discussion about outcomes and patient expectations. Although only a relative contraindication (see **Box 1**) we have had 1 patient who although a large osteophyte was removed by minimally invasive cheilectomy and did not have a good outcome because her preexisting panarticular osteoarthritis progressed relentlessly and quickly into a very painful and very stiff joint.

SUMMARY

Minimally invasive cheilectomy results in excellent patient reported outcomes of pain relief and early return to function. Very few if any significant complications are reported in the literature. Patient satisfaction seems to be a positive indicator for the use of minimally invasive cheilectomy, which may well become the gold standard treatment in the near future. Patients and surgeons need to be aware of the limitations of cheilectomy in the presence of advanced articular surface osteoarthritis as shown clinically by a positive grind test.

REFERENCES

1. Harrison T, Fawzy E, Dinah F, et al. Prospective assessment of dorsal cheilectomy for hallux rigidus using a patient-reported outcome score. J Foot Ankle Surg 2010; 49(3):232–7.
2. Morgan S, Jones C, Palmer S. Minimally invasive cheilectomy (MIS): functional outcome and comparison with open cheilectomy. J Bone Joint Surg Br 2012;94-B-(Suppl XLI):93.

Percutaneous Surgery for Mild to Moderate Hallux Valgus

Peter Lam, MB BS (Hons), FRACS[a,*], Moses Lee, MD[b], Jerry Xing, MD[a], Martin Di Nallo, MD[a]

KEYWORDS

• Hallux valgus • Percutaneous • Minimally invasive • Chevron • Akin

KEY POINTS

- Available data suggest that patients who undergo percutaneous chevron-Akin osteotomies have less pain at follow-up, greater (or at least comparable to open techniques such as scarf osteotomy) correction of hallux valgus angle, and a shorter operation time compared with open osteotomies.
- Stable fixation of the chevron osteotomy allows early full weight bearing and mobilization of the first metatarsophalangeal joint.
- The 3 most important steps in the surgery technique are reduction of the first metatarsal head after translation to prevent dorsal or plantar displacement or angulation, accurate positioning of the proximal first metatarsal fixation screw to provide stability to the fixation, and removal of the dorsomedial prominence of the first metatarsal head.

INTRODUCTION

Hallux valgus is a combination of valgus and pronation deformity of the big toe along with varus positioning of the first metatarsal. It is a common problem often associated with patient dysfunction. Pain can be felt over the medial eminence due to inflammation of the overlying bursa, irritation of the dorsal cutaneous nerve, or be associated with deformities of the lesser toes. Symptomatic patients who have failed conservative measures are candidates for surgery. Over the years, there have been more than 150 different techniques[1] described for surgical correction of hallux valgus. One of the more popular procedures in Australia is the scarf-Akin osteotomy. A 2004 Cochrane Review did not favor any one procedure compared with another.[2] There

The authors have nothing to disclose.

[a] Orthopaedic and Arthritis Specialist Centre, Level 2, 445 Victoria Avenue, Chatswood, Sydney 2067, New South Wales, Australia; [b] Department of Orthopedic Surgery, Yonsei Sarang Hospital, 478-3, Bangbae-dong, Seocho-gu, Seoul, Korea
* Corresponding author.
E-mail address: admin@peterlam.com.au

is a general consensus in treatment, however, that distal osteotomies are reserved for mild to moderate deformities whereas proximal osteotomies are more powerful at correcting severe deformities. The hallux valgus angle (HVA), intermetatarsal angle (IMA), distal metatarsophalangeal joint congruity, and presence of arthritis are factors used to determine the optimal treatment procedure. Open bunion correction is generally effective but can be associated with significant postoperative pain and disability.

Percutaneous and minimally invasive surgery have garnered attention in orthopedics due to the potential for smaller scars, less postoperative pain, quicker recovery, decreased rehabilitation times, and reduced risk of infection and wound complications.[3,4] Its applications in hallux valgus correction was first introduced in the 1970s and 1980s.[5] It has since evolved into endoscopic, minimum-incision, and percutaneous techniques. Minimum-incision surgery involves correcting the deformity through small incisions that still allow direct visualizations of the osseous procedures. In contrast, percutaneous surgeries are performed through the smallest possible incisions without a direct view and using tactile sensation combined with image intensification. Over the past decade, there has been a growing interest in percutaneous techniques for hallux valgus correction especially in Europe. First-generation percutaneous technique was described by Isham[5] in which there was no internal fixation following the osteotomy.

The second-generation technique was a distal transverse osteotomy of the first metatarsal stabilized with an axial wire.[6–12] Third-generation technique with screw fixation has added extra stability.[13,14] The authors present our preferred method of percutaneous hallux valgus correction based on the percutaneous modified chevron-Akin (PECA) technique described by Vernois and Redfern.[15] Three recent review articles concluded there was not enough evidence to recommend minimally invasive surgery compared with traditional open surgery.[16–18] This is because there has been limited published literature on percutaneous procedures and most publications are case series without control or comparison groups. To date, there is no published prospective randomized trial comparing PECA osteotomies and scarf-Akin osteotomies for the correction of hallux valgus.

INDICATIONS OR CONTRAINDICATIONS

The authors' indication for the use of the percutaneous procedure is a reducible hallux valgus when the HVA is up to 45° and the IMA is up to 20°. The procedure can be performed in patients with increased distal metatarsal angle, metatarsus adductus, and in cases of mild asymptomatic degenerative arthritis of the first metatarsophalangeal joint. In patients with mild to moderate arthritis of the first metatarsophalangeal joint, the joint needs to be passively correctable in the transverse plane in order for it to be suitable for bunion correction surgery.

Contraindications include severe deformity with IMA greater than 20°, moderately severe degenerative disease of the first metatarsophalangeal joint, lesser degree of arthritis in which the first metatarsophalangeal joint is not reducible, and severe instability of the first tarsometatarsal joint.

SURGICAL TECHNIQUE

The procedure can be performed under general or regional anesthesia with or without tourniquet. The authors' preference is general anesthesia with the use of a thigh tourniquet. The patient is positioned supine with the feet over the end of the operating table (**Fig. 1**). The image intensifier (preferably mini C-arm) is introduced from the right

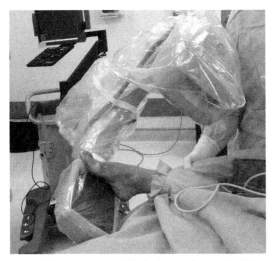

Fig. 1. The patient is positioned supine with feet over the end of the operating table to allow easy access to the image intensifier.

side, perpendicular to the long axis of the operating table (see **Fig. 1**). We perform bilateral surgery on the right foot first to reduce the risk of contamination of the right foot from the image intensifier.

The dorsal and plantar outline of the first metatarsal is made (**Fig. 2**). Using a 15 blade, 3 mm incisions are made over the midpoint (dorsoplantar of first metatarsal head) at the medial aspect of the first metatarsophalangeal joint (marked A in **Fig. 2**), midpoint (dorsoplantar of first metatarsal) at the base of the flare of the medial eminence (distal diaphyseal-metaphyseal junction) (marked B in **Fig. 2**), and a 5 mm incision is made just distal to the medial aspect of the first tarsometatarsal joint (marked C in **Fig. 2**). The chevron osteotomy is made using a 2 × 20 mm burr. The burr is introduced through incision B. The initial insertion of the burr into the first metatarsal will form the apex of the chevron cut. The burr will remove approximately 3 mm of bone. If the burr is directed perpendicular to the axis of the second metatarsal (**Fig. 3**), as the metatarsal head is displaced laterally it will displace the head fragment

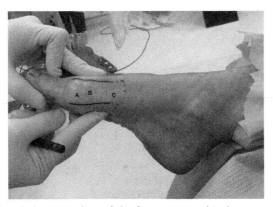

Fig. 2. The dorsal and plantar outline of the first metatarsal is drawn.

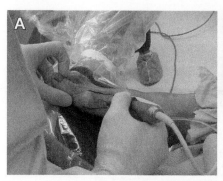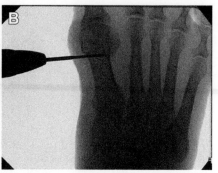

Fig. 3. (*A*) Placement of the burr through portal B. (*B*) The burr to cut the modified chevron osteotomy is directed perpendicular to the axis of the second metatarsal.

distally by about 3 mm. This will counteract the effect of the burr shortening and thus prevent any significant overall shortening of the first metatarsal. The burr is also directed in a plantar direction of approximately 10°. However, in patients with a long first metatarsal, it may be desirable to direct the burr more proximally to allow shortening of the first metatarsal. The dorsal limb of the osteotomy is performed next, then the plantar limb. For the plantar cut, we direct the burr to aim for the skin of the heel in preference for a short plantar limb. After the osteotomy is completed, we insert a 1.6 mm K wire from the medial base of the first metatarsal distally (through the incision marked C in **Fig. 2**), in the midaxis of the metatarsal bone, and perforate the far cortex of the distal first metatarsal so the wire exits the bone approximately 1 cm proximal to the osteotomy (**Fig. 4**). We then withdraw the 1.6 K wire and insert the 1 mm guidewire. We prefer this technique because the current 1 mm guidewire is too flexible to allow easily reproducible placement of the wire for the proximal screw. The placement of the proximal fixation screw is extremely important because this allows stable fixation of the osteotomy. The placement of the 1.6 K wire in the midaxial line (**Fig. 5**) means the wire will exit the lateral cortex but, if the wire is directed in a too plantarly direction, the wire can exit through the osteotomy but appear to go through the lateral cortex on the image intensifier. If this happens, stable fixation is not achieved and the head will

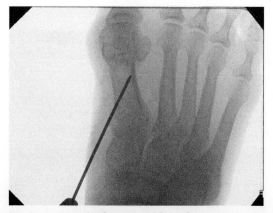

Fig. 4. The 1.6 K wire aims to exit the far cortex of the first metatarsal approximately 1 cm proximal to the osteotomy.

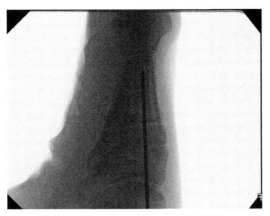

Fig. 5. Lateral image to confirm 1.6 K wire is in the midaxial line.

redisplace medially, resulting in loss of correction (**Fig. 6**). A 2 mm diameter guidewire is inserted through the incision A as shown in **Fig. 2**, through the osteotomy into the shaft of the first metatarsal to allow displacement of the metatarsal head. The reduction maneuver is important. The first step is to use the right hand to make sure the head is in alignment in the lateral plane (**Fig. 7**). This prevents plantar or dorsal displacement, or tilt of the first metatarsal head. The second step is to use the left hand with the aid of the 2 mm wire to displace the head laterally (**Fig. 8**). The third step is to correct the pronation of the metatarsal head (**Fig. 9**). Once this is achieved, advance the 1 mm guidewire through the far cortex of the first metatarsal into the head (**Fig. 10**). The screw is then inserted. If there were increased distal metatarsal articular angle (DMAA), correct this by applying a gentle varus force to the head as the screw is inserted into the head fragment (**Fig. 11**). A second metatarsal screw is inserted to provide rotational stability and strength to the construct. It is important to obtain internal oblique views of the foot to confirm the head of the screws are completely engaged in the bone. This is because the screw head may appear completely engaged on the anteroposterior view but may still be proud. If this occurs, the prominent screw can cause irritation and possibly require its removal at a later date. The Akin osteotomy is then performed with a 2 × 12 mm burr and this osteotomy is fixed with a cannulated screw introduced from the medial base of the distal phalanx (**Fig. 12**). A distal soft tissue release is performed with insertion of a beaver blade from the dorsum of the first metatarsophalangeal joint just lateral to the extensor hallucis longus tendon. The blade then divides the lateral plantar plate and the lateral sesamoid phalangeal ligament. Image intensifier control is used with each step to confirm satisfactory correction and fixation of the osteotomies. Through incision B, as seen in **Fig. 2**, a curved periosteal elevator is used to puncture the medial capsule just distal to the capsular attachment on the medial eminence. A 3.1 mm wedge burr is used to remove the medial prominence. The adequacy of the removal is confirmed on the image intensifier (**Fig. 13**). We also use the 3.1 mm wedge burr to remove any medial prominence of the proximal first metatarsal at the site of the osteotomy. The dressing includes nonadherent dressing (such as Adaptic [Johnson & Johnson]), dry gauze, soft band, and crepe bandage. Postoperatively, the patient is allowed to bear full weight as tolerated in a flat postoperative shoe for 2 weeks. We request and encourage patients to walk with their foot flat on the ground rather than on the lateral border of the foot. The patients are advised to walk with the aid of crutches for up to 2 weeks after the operation. We

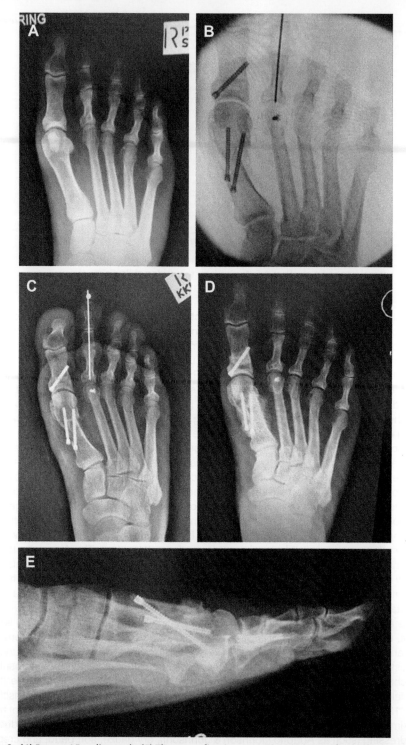

Fig. 6. (*A*) Pre-op AP radiograph. (*B*) The screw fixation on AP image intensifier looked satisfactory. *C* and *D* 6 and 12 week post op radiograph show loss of reduction and fixation. (*E*) The lateral radiograph showed the loss of fixation was due to the proximal 1st metatarsal screw been placed in too plantar a direction resulting in the screw passing through the osteotomy. This did not provide rigid fixation and resulted in loss of reduction of the metatarsal head. (*Courtesy of* Todd Gothelf, MD, Kingswood, Australia.)

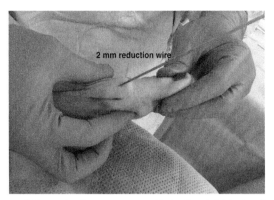

Fig. 7. The first step of the reduction maneuver. Note the right index finger lifting up the first metatarsal head to ensure the first metatarsal head is reduced in the lateral plane.

request the patient to elevate the foot or feet as much as possible in the first 10 days after the operation to reduce the degree of foot swelling. We review the patients 10 to 14 days after the operation. We start gentle plantarflexion stretching exercises of the first metatarsophalangeal joint after 2 weeks to help regain the joint motion and scar massage to desensitize the scars. We place the foot in a bunion sleeve (**Fig. 14**). This is worn with a pair of firm sports socks during the day only for 6 to 12 weeks. The authors believe this helps with the shortening of the medial capsule without performing a formal capsulorrhaphy. We advise against wearing the bunion sleeve on its own without a sock because it can lead to a hallux varus alignment (**Fig. 15**). We allow patients to wear a pair of sneakers with a straight medial last after 2 weeks. Standard weight-bearing radiographs are performed at 6-weeks and 6-months postoperatively (**Figs. 16–18**). To date, the senior author (PL) have performed more than 1500 hallux valgus corrections with this technique and have not experienced any nonunion or avascular necrosis.

METHOD

A prospective randomized review of 51 subjects[19] undergoing surgical correction of the hallux was done, with the subjects randomized to 2 groups, 1 treated with

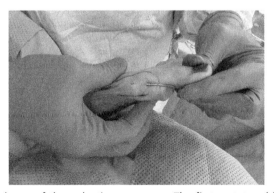

Fig. 8. The second step of the reduction maneuver. The first metatarsal head is displaced laterally with the aid of the 2 mm wire. The right index finger is preventing redisplacement of the first metatarsal head during this maneuver.

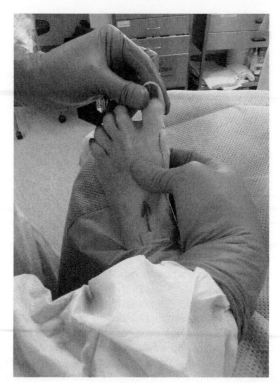

Fig. 9. The third step of the reduction maneuver. The first metatarsal head pronation is corrected before advancing the 1.1 mm guidewire into the first metatarsal head.

scarf-Akin (scarf) osteotomies and the other with the PECA osteotomies. Outcomes measures included American Orthopedic Foot and Ankle Society (AOFAS) Hallux-Metatarsophalangeal-Interphalangeal Score, visual analog pain score (pain VAS), HVA, and 1 to 2 IMA. Outcomes were measured preoperatively, and then 6 and

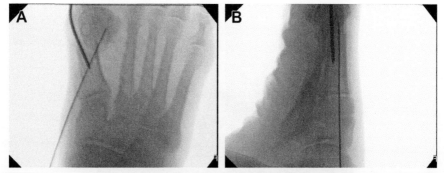

Fig. 10. (*A*) Final confirmation anteroposterior radiograph of the reduction and positioning of the wire before drilling and insertion of the proximal first metatarsal fixation screw. (*B*) Final confirmation lateral radiograph of the reduction and positioning of the wire before drilling and insertion of the proximal first metatarsal fixation screw.

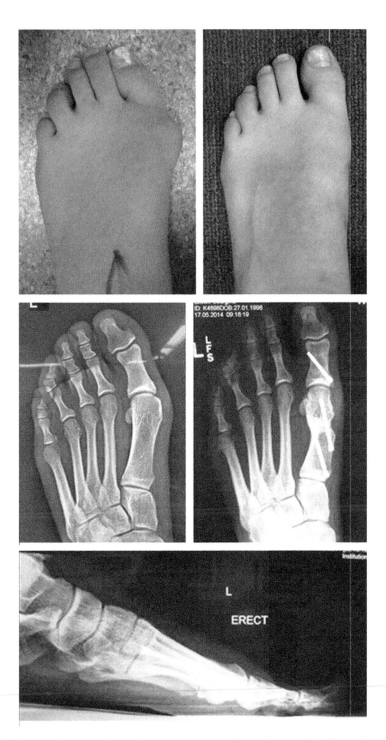

Fig. 11. Preoperative and 6 months postoperative of a patient with hallux valgus, with increased DMAA. *A (top left)* Pre-op clinical; *B (top right)* 6 month post-op clinical; *C (Middle left)* Pre-op AP radiograph; *D (Middle right)* 6 month post-op AP radiograph; *E (Bottom)* 6 month post-op lateral radiograph, note the proximal first metatarsal screw is in the mid axial line on the lateral radiograph.

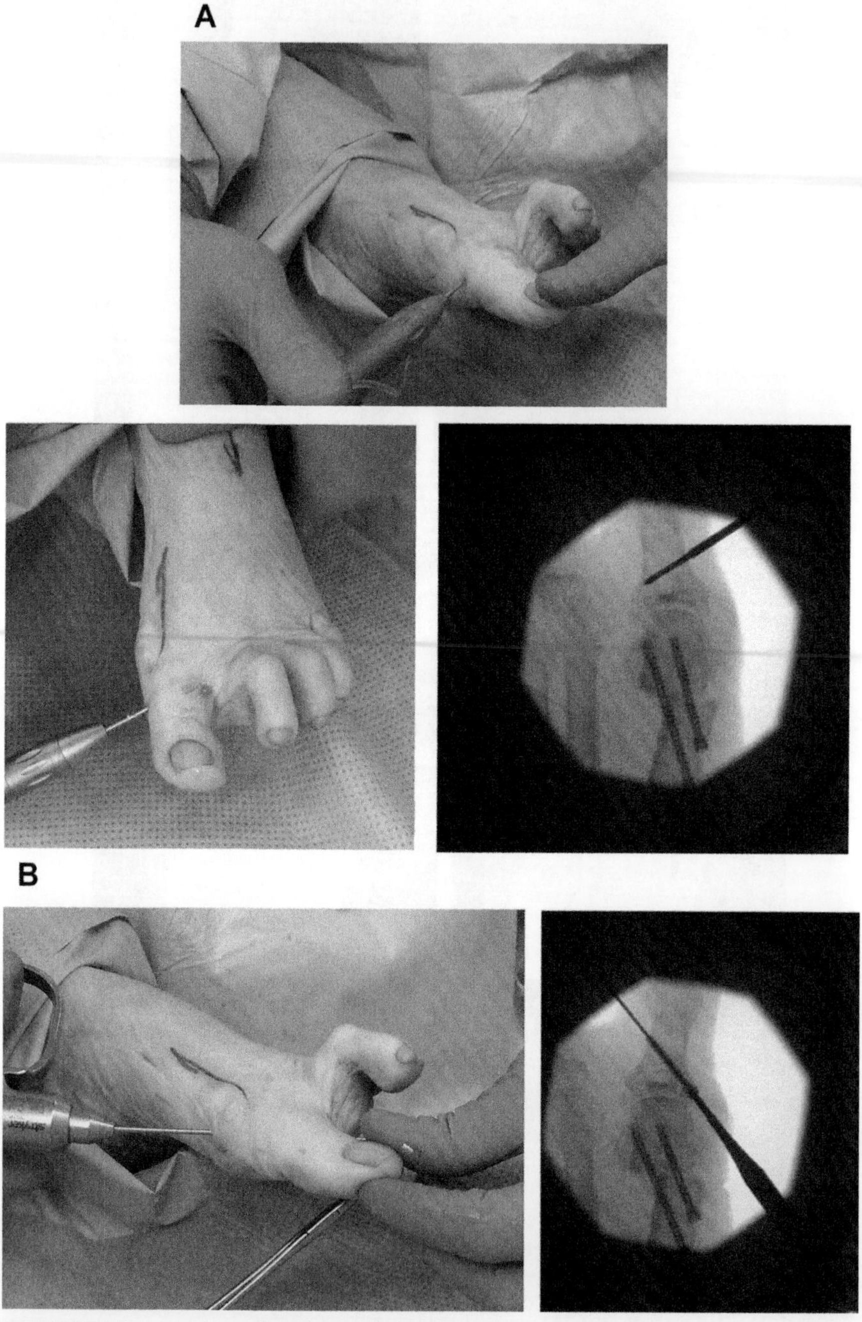

Fig. 12. (*A*) The burr is introduced perpendicular to the axis of the toe. (*B*) Once the burr has perforated the medial cortex then the burr is directed proximally to allow an oblique Akin osteotomy. (*C*) (*middle right*) the position of the burr is confirmed with the image intensifier. *D* (*bottom left*) The placement of the guidewire and screw through portal A (see **Fig. 2**) is directed approximately perpendicular to the oblique osteotomy. *E* (*bottom right*) The placement of the guide wire and screw is confirmed on the image intensifier.

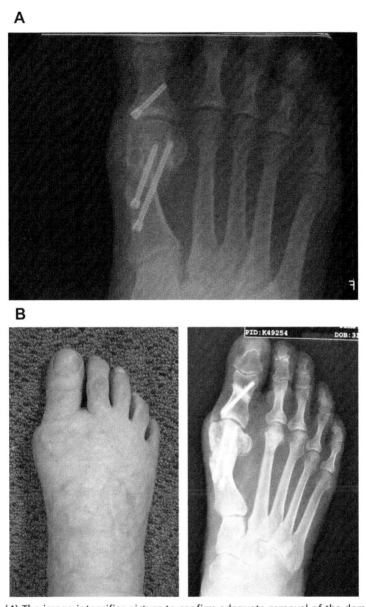

Fig. 13. (*A*) The image intensifier picture to confirm adequate removal of the dorsomedial eminence at the first metatarsal head. (*B*) 12 months clinical and radiograph showing the residual bunion, partly due to not resecting the dorsomedial eminence at the time of the bunion correction surgery. *B1* (*bottom left*) and *B2* (*bottom right*) 12 months clinical and AP radiograph showing the residual bunion, partly due to not resecting the dorsomedial eminence at the time of the bunion correction surgery.

26 weeks postoperatively, with pain VAS also at day 1 and 2 weeks. The radiographic outcomes parameters were measured using weight-bearing radiographs.

RESULTS

There were 26 (3 men) subjects with 27 feet (1 bilateral) who underwent scarf-Akin procedures and 25 subjects (2 men) with 33 feet (8 bilateral) who had PECA procedures. The

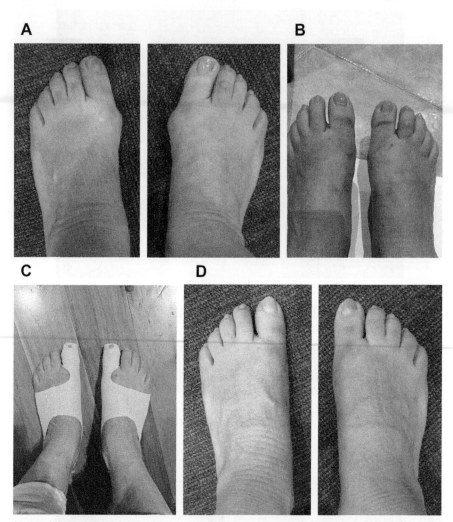

Fig. 14. (*A*) Preoperative left hallux valgus and preoperative right hallux valgus. (*B*) 2-weeks postoperative appearance. (*C*) 2-weeks postoperative appearance in bunion sleeve. (*D*) 3-months postoperative appearance left foot and right foot. *A1* (*top left*) Preoperative left hallux valgus. *A2* (*top middle*) Preoperative right hallux valgus. *D1* (*bottom middle*) 3-months postoperative appearance of the left foot and *D2* (*bottom right*) right foot.

scarf group had a higher mean age of 58 years (95% CI 54–63) than the PECA group mean age of 47 years (41–53; P = .004). By 26 weeks, the AOFAS score improved from 58 (54–62) to 83 (83–87; $P<.001$) in the scarf group and 61 (58–65) to 89 (87–91; $P<.001$) in the PECA group. This change from baseline was not significantly different between surgery groups (P = .56). By 26 weeks, the HVA decreased from 31° (27–35) to 10.1° (8.2–12.0) in the Scarf group ($P<.001$) and from 31° (29–33) to 7.6° (6.4–8.9) in the PECA group ($P<.001$). If corrected for the difference in the age of subjects between groups, PECA surgery is 3.4° (−6.6 to −0.3) better than scarf surgery (P = .033).

The IMA decreased from an average of 15.7° (14.3–17.1) to 7.6° (6.7–8.5) in the scarf group by 26 weeks ($P<.001$) and from 15.6° (14.6–16.8) to 6.4° (5.6–7.3) in the PECA group ($P<.001$), with the difference between surgical groups not significant (P = .25).

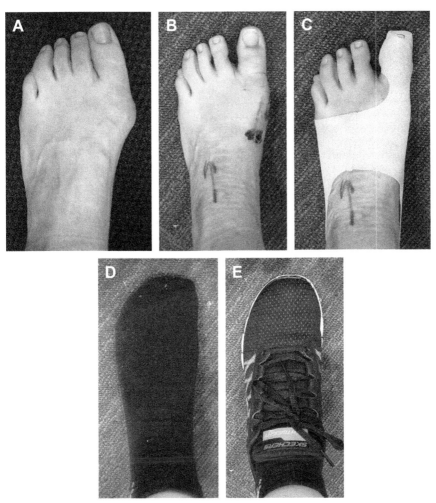

Fig. 15. (*A*) Preoperative left hallux valgus. (*B*) 2-weeks postoperative appearance. (*C*) 2-weeks postoperative appearance in bunion sleeve. Note the bunion sleeve is pulling the hallux into varus alignment. (*D*) Wearing firm sports sock to maintain correct alignment of hallux. (*E*) Wearing sneaker with straight medial last at 2-weeks postoperative with the bunion sleeve and firm sports sock.

The combined scar length was significantly shorter in the PECA group at 24.2 (20.6–27.8) mm compared with 108 (106–110) mm for the scarf group (*P*<.001). There was no incidence of dorsal or plantar malunion in the PECA group. The operative time was also shorter in the PECA group at 29.7 (27.8–31.6) minutes compared with 33.7 (31.3–36.1) minutes for the scarf group (*P* = .009). The average radiation screen time was 31.6 (27.9–35.3) seconds in the PECA group. The pain VAS was significantly lower for PECA than scarf surgery at day 1 (*P*<.001), day 2 (*P*<.001), and 6 weeks (*P* = .004) but not 26 weeks. There were no complications in terms of infection, wound breakdown, chronic regional pain syndrome, or nonunion of the osteotomies. In the scarf group, there were 2 subjects who developed mild second metatarsalgia postoperative. The metatarsalgia settled with orthotic treatment and further surgery was not required.

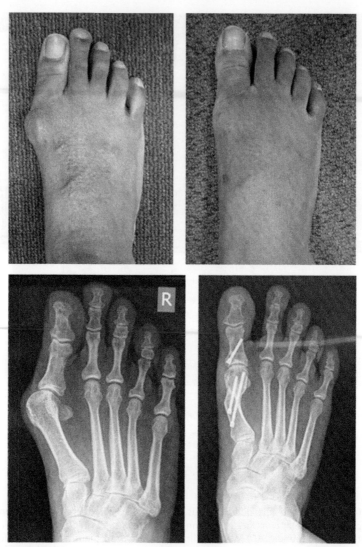

Fig. 16. The preoperative and 6-months postoperative of patient with moderate hallux valgus. *A* (*top left*) Preoperative clinical appearance of moderate right hallux valgus. *B* (*top right*) 6-months postoperative appearance. *C* (*bottom left*) Preoperative AP radiograph. *D* (*bottom right*) 6-months postoperative AP radiograph showing correction of 1st metatarsal head subluxation.

One of these subjects also complained of increased depth from dorsal to plantar of the foot after the surgery. In the PECA group, 6 required screw removal. The incidence of screw removal has been almost eliminated by the use of the internal oblique view to confirm the screw is fully engaged in the bone at the time of screw insertion.

DISCUSSION

This study showed significantly less pain at follow-up, greater correction of HVA and a shorter operation time in the PECA subject group, as well as the expected shorter scar

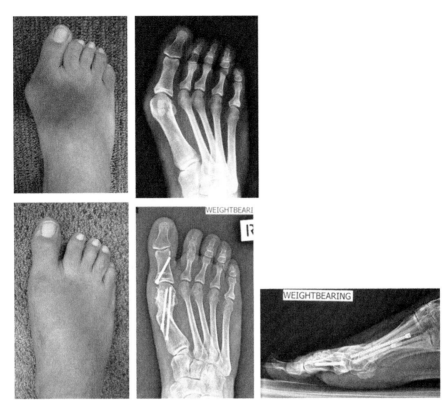

Fig. 17. The preoperative and 6-months postoperative clinical and radiographs of correction of hallux valgus with metatarsus adductus. *A (top left)* Preoperative clinical appearance of right hallux valgus with metatarsus adductus. *B (top right)* Preoperative AP radiograph. *C (bottom left)* 6-months postoperative appearance. *D (bottom middle)* 6-months postoperative AP radiograph. *E (bottom right)* 6 month post-op lateral radiograph, note the proximal first metatarsal screw is in the mid axial line on the lateral radiograph.

length. IMA and AOFAS score were not different between surgeries. The limitation of this study is the short follow-up. An endeavor will be made to report the longer term results in a few years.

The percutaneous chevron-Akin procedure has been demonstrated to have minimal risk to neurovascular and tendon injury in a cadaveric study by Dhukaram.[20]

There is sparse literature on the first-generation technique in which there is no internal fixation. In 1991, Weinberger and colleagues[21] published 301 cases with 204 subjects. The HVA improved from 26 to 7.5. Complications included superficial infection 3.65%, second metatarsal stress fracture 2.32%, and delayed union 1.32%. Bauer and colleagues[22] reported on 104 cases with 2 year follow-up. The HVA improved from 30° to 15° and the IMA reduced from 14° to 11°. However, complications included 4 1st metatarsal (M1) and 5 proximal phalanx (P1) lateral cortical fractures, not requiring revision surgery. Six cases of DMAA overcorrection, 2 painful stiff first metatarsophalangeal joint with global stiffness, 2 cases of chronic regional pain syndrome, and 2 recurrences.

Most of literature reports on the use of percutaneous osteotomy with K wire fixation (second-generation). The K wire fixation does not provide rigid stable fixation and this may allow potential for dorsal and plantar displacement of the metatarsal head. Most papers did not report on the dorsal or plantar displacement. Magnan and colleagues[8]

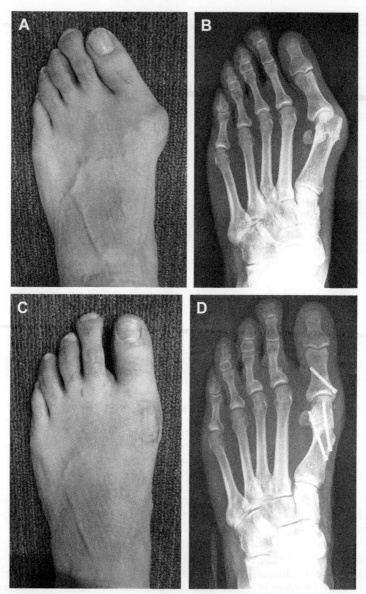

Fig. 18. The preoperative and 6-months postoperative clinical and radiographs of correction of hallux valgus with lateral deviation of the lesser toes. Importantly, sometimes associated lateral plane deformity of the second and third toes needs to be corrected at the time of the bunion correction surgery. (*A*) (*top left*) Preoperative clinical appearance of left hallux valgus with moderately severe HVA and lateral deviation of the lesser toes. (*B*) (*top right*) Preoperative AP radiograph. (*C*) (*bottom left*) 6-months postoperative appearance, it is important to note that sometimes associated lateral plane deformity of the second and third toes needs to be corrected at the same time. (*D*) (*bottom right*) 6-months postoperative AP radiograph.

reported 49% had plantar displacement (mainly plantar translation with some degree of plantar angulation) and 12% had dorsiflexion (mainly angular deformity). Enan and colleagues[23] reported 47.3% had plantar displacement (mainly plantar translation with some degree of plantar angulation) and 8.3% had dorsal displacement (mainly angular deformity). Iannò and colleagues[24] reported 3.5% dorsal angulation and 1.2% had plantar angulation. The use of wire fixation may also be associated with a higher risk of infection. The incidence of superficial infection has been reported to range from 0% to 8.5%, deep infection from 0% to 4.1%, and pressure sore from the K wire from 0% to 12.8%.[6–12,23,24] Avascular necrosis was reported by Iannò[24] (3/ 85) and Kadakia and colleagues[12] (1/13). Kadakia and colleagues[12] planned a prospective study but they had to stop the study after 13 cases due to unacceptable rate of complication, including malunion, nonunion, recurrence, osteonecrosis, and infection. This may be because their study included their learning curve. The consensus of the published literature is that percutaneous distal first metatarsal osteotomy allows good correction of moderate hallux valgus deformity. The authors found 3 published comparative studies, 2 comparing PECA and scarf osteotomy,[25,26] and 1 comparing percutaneous distal metatarsal osteotomy and open distal chevron osteotomy.[27] All 3 studies used K wire fixation in the percutaneous distal first metatarsal osteotomy group. The 3 studies showed good radiological result with no statistically significant difference between the groups. For correction of HVA and IMA, the operative time was significantly shorter in the percutaneous groups: Giannini and colleagues,[26] 3 minutes versus 17 minutes (scarf); Maffulli and colleagues,[25] 19 minutes versus 42 minutes (scarf); and Radwan and Mansour,[27] 51 min versus 58 min (chevron).

There is a paucity of published papers in the English-speaking literature on the use of screw fixation (third-generation) in percutaneous distal metatarsal osteotomy. In 2011, Vernois[28] reported on his early experience using a combination of K wire and screw fixation. He reported HVA decreased from 37° to 10. There were 3 recurrences that required revision surgery. In 2014, Brogan and colleagues[13] reported on the use of a combination of wire and screw fixation in 45 feet. Mean HVA decreased from 30.54° to 10.41° and mean IMA decreased from 14.55° to 7.11°. Two subjects complained of prominent screws and 1 required removal of the screw. In 2011, Redfern and colleagues[29] reported on his early experience of using a single-screw fixation alone in 30 feet with average of 3 months follow-up. There were no cases of infection, 2 cases of chronic regional pain syndrome, and 2 screws required removal.

The authors believe it is important to understand that percutaneous distal first metatarsal osteotomy relates to the skin incision or approach to performing the osteotomy. Once the osteotomy is performed with the burr, the general principles of lateral translation and need for rigid internal fixation is similar to other procedures, such as with open scarf and chevron osteotomies. Without adequate lateral translation to reduce the IMA and stable internal fixation, the surgery is doomed to fail. The authors believe 2-screw fixation provides the most stable construct for the fixation in percutaneous distal first metatarsal osteotomy. This should reduce the risk of loss of correction, resulting in recurrent hallux valgus or transfer metatarsalgia.

In terms of the technical side of the percutaneous distal first metatarsal osteotomy, the authors believe the 3 most important steps are:

1. To make sure the first metatarsal head is reduced in the lateral plane when translating the metatarsal head so that the head is not displaced or angulated dorsally or plantarly. The surgeon must be aware that the displacement technique (see previous discussion) has a tendency to cause plantar displacement or angulation.

2. Insertion of the guidewire for the proximal screw is in the line of the axis of the first metatarsal in the lateral plane. Do not allow the guidewire to penetrate the lateral (far) cortex of the first metatarsal until the correct alignment is attained. If the wire is too plantarly directed, the wire is likely to miss the lateral (far) cortex and go through the osteotomy or the guidewire may penetrate the lateral (far) cortex too close to the plantar aspect of the osteotomy. If the latter situation happens, the screw may break the bony bridge as it is inserted and this will result in the loss of fixation. If the proximal screw is placed in the proximal medial cortex and passes through the distal lateral cortex (proximal to the osteotomy) before it enters the metatarsal head fragment, the metatarsal head cannot displace. This is the ideal situation leading to stable fixation. The current screw that is available for the proximal screw fixation is good but not ideal, especially in the patient who is heavier or has larger feet. Further work needs to done to design a better screw for these patients.

3. Remove the dorsomedial prominence of the metatarsal head. If this is not removed, the patient can still see and feel the dorsomedial prominence, leading to reduced patient satisfaction after surgery.

SUMMARY

The available literature suggests the PECA technique, in particular the third-generation using screw fixation, is a safe and reliable technique for the correction of hallux valgus. It provides comparable correction of HVA and IMA with no increase in complication compared with open techniques. PECA technique has the added advantages of shorter operative time and shorter scar length and is associated with a higher level of patient satisfaction.

REFERENCES

1. Helal B. Surgery for adolescent hallux valgus. Clin Orthop 1981;157:50–63.
2. Ferrari J, Higgins JP, Prior TD. Interventions for treating hallux valgus (abducto-valgus) and bunions. Cochrane Database Syst Rev 2004;(1):CD000964.
3. Longo UG, Papapietro N, Maffulli N, et al. Thoracoscopy for minimally invasive thoracic spine surgery. Orthop Clin North Am 2009;40:459–64.
4. Khanna A, Gougoulias N, Longo UG, et al. Minimally invasive total knee arthroplasty: a systematic review. Orthop Clin North Am 2009;40:479–89.
5. Isham S. The Reverdin-Isham procedure for the correction of hallux abducto valgus. A distal metatarsal osteotomy procedure. Clin Podiatr Med Surg 1991;8:81–94.
6. Portaluri M. Hallux valgus correction by the method of Bösch: a clinical evaluation. Foot Ankle Clin 2000;5:499–511.
7. Sanna P, Ruiu GA. Percutaneous distal osteotomy of the first metatarsal (PDO) for the surgical treatment of hallux valgus. Chir Organi Mov 2005;90:365–9.
8. Magnan B, Pezzè L, Rossi N, et al. Percutaneous distal metatarsal osteotomy for correction of hallux valgus. J Bone Joint Surg Am 2005;87:1191–9.
9. Bösch P, Wanke S, Legenstein R. Hallux valgus correction by the method of Bösch: a new technique with a seven-to-ten-year follow-up. Foot Ankle Clin 2000;5:485–98.
10. Giannini S, Ceccarelli F, Bevoni R, et al. Hallux valgus surgery: the minimally invasive bunion correction. Tech Foot Ankle Surg 2003;2:11–20.
11. Maffulli N, Oliva F, Coppola C, et al. Minimally invasive hallux valgus correction: a technical note and a feasibility study. J Surg Orthop Adv 2005;14(4):193–8.

12. Kadakia AR, Smerek JP, Myerson MS. Radiographic results after percutaneous distal metatarsal osteotomy for correction of hallux valgus deformity. Foot Ankle Int 2007;28:355–60.
13. Brogan K, Voller T, Gee C, et al. Third-generation minimally invasive correction of hallux valgus: technique and early outcomes. Int Orthop 2014;38:2115–21.
14. Redfern D, Perera AM. Minimally invasive osteotomies. Foot Ankle Clin N Am 2014;19:181–9.
15. Vernois J, Redfern DJ. Percutaneous Chevron; the union of classic stable fixed approach and percutaneous technique. Fuss & Sprunggelenk 2013;11(2):70–5.
16. Roukis TS. Percutaneous and minimum incision metatarsal osteotomies: a systematic review. J Foot Ankle Surg 2009;48:380–7.
17. Maffulli N, Longo UG, Marinozzi A, et al. Hallux valgus: effectiveness and safety of minimally invasive surgery. A systematic review. Br Med Bull 2001;97:149–67.
18. Trnka HJ, Krenn S, Schuh R. Minimally invasive hallux valgus surgery: a critical review of the evidence. Int Orthop 2013;37(9):1731–5.
19. Lam P, Wines A, Smith MM, et al. Prospective randomised review of hallux valgus correction comparing scarf/Akin osteotomies and percutaneous Chevron/Akin osteotomies. Paper presented at AOFAS Summer Meeting. Chicago IL, September 19–23, 2014.
20. Dhukaram V, Chapman AP. Minimally invasive forefoot surgery: a cadaveric study. Foot Ankle Int 2012;33(12):1139–43.
21. Weinberger BH, Fulp JM, Falstrom P, et al. Retrospective evaluation of percutaneous bunionectomies and distal osteotomies without internal fixation. Clin Podiatr Med Surg 1991;8:111–36.
22. Bauer T, Biau D, Lortat-Jacob A, et al. Percutaneous hallux valgus correction using the Reverdin-Isham osteotomy. Orthop Traumatol Surg Res 2010;96(4):407–16.
23. Enan A, Abo-Hegy M, Seif H. Early results of distal metatarsal osteotomy through minimally invasive approach for mild-to-moderate hallux valgus. Acta Orthop Belg 2010;76:526–35.
24. Iannò B, Familiari F, De Gori M, et al. Midterm results and complications after minimally invasive distal metatarsal osteotomy for treatment of hallux valgus. Foot Ankle Int 2013;34:969–77.
25. Maffulli N, Longo UG, Oliva F, et al. Bosch osteotomy and scarf osteotomy for hallux valgus correction. Orthop Clin North Am 2009;40:515–24.
26. Giannini S, Cavallo M, Faldini C, et al. The SERI distal metatarsal osteotomy and Scarf osteotomy provide similar correction of hallux valgus. Clin Orthop Relat Res 2013;471:2305–11.
27. Radwan YA, Mansour AM. Percutaneous distal metatarsal osteotomy versus distal chevron osteotomy for correction of mild-to-moderate hallux valgus deformity. Arch Orthop Trauma Surg 2012;132:1539–46.
28. Vernois J. The treatment of the hallux valgus with a percutaneous Chevron osteotomy. J Bone Joint Surg (Br) 2011;93-B(Supp IV). p. 482.
29. Redfern D, Gill I, Harris M. Early experience with a minimally invasive modified Chevron and Akin osteotomy for correction of hallux valgus. J Bone Joint Surg (Br) 2011;93-B(Supp IV). p. 482.

Percutaneous Surgery for Severe Hallux Valgus

Joel Vernois, MD[a,b,*], David J. Redfern, FRCS (Tr&Orth)[c]

KEYWORDS

- Hallux valgus • Percutaneous • Distal chevron • Proximal basal osteotomy • MICA

KEY POINTS

- Severe hallux valgus is a challenge to treat.
- Chevron and basal osteotomy percutaneous procedures have been recently described.
- A basal osteotomy is a well-known surgery for severe deformity and the chevron osteotomy is often used for mild to moderate deformity.
- Percutaneous techniques are adequate procedures to correct all deformities. Surgeons need appropriate cadaveric training to gain experience.

INTRODUCTION

The definition of severe hallux valgus is multifactorial. Assessment with multiple measures and the shape of the forefoot define the severity of the deformity, whereas certain measures and the reducibility of the deformity define the technical possibilities. When a distal classic chevron osteotomy is not possible, a proximal osteotomy is the solution. Typically, the severity of the deformity is determined with the intermetatarsal angle (IMA or M1M2) angle in an anteroposterior (AP) view of a full weight bearing radiograph. Unfortunately, this angle does not take into account the length of the first metatarsal and the width of the head of the metatarsal, which are both the key in surgical planning.

The authors prefer to assess the deformity clinically. The space between the first and second metatarsal head is evaluated and compared with the size of the first metatarsal head. If the width is enough to fill the intermetatarsal space, a distal modified chevron osteotomy can correct the deformity. If not, a proximal osteotomy is the solution.

Since 2002, percutaneous surgery has been promoted in Europe by the Groupe de Recherche et d'Etude en Chirurgie Mini Invasive du Pied (GRECMIP; www.grecmip.org). Initially created by an group of French surgeons due to their

The authors have nothing to disclose.
[a] Sussex Orthopaedic Treatment Centre, Haywards Heath RH16 4EY, UK; [b] ICP, 8 Lacepede street, 75005 Paris, France; [c] London Foot and Ankle Centre, Hospital of St. John and St. Elizabeth, 60 Grove End Road, London NW8 9NH, UK
* Corresponding author.
E-mail address: joel.vernois@sfr.fr

Foot Ankle Clin N Am 21 (2016) 479–493
http://dx.doi.org/10.1016/j.fcl.2016.04.002
1083-7515/16/$ – see front matter © 2016 Elsevier Inc. All rights reserved.

foot.theclinics.com

interest in arthroscopy and minimally invasive surgery of the foot and ankle, the GRECMIP is now an international group of surgeons developing and teaching arthroscopy and percutaneous surgery. This group developed a percutaneous chevron surgery for the treatment of mild to moderate deformity that was presented in Arcachon, France, in June 2007, at the French Foot and Ankle Association.[1] With a modification of the fixation, minimally invasive chevron and Akin (MICA) osteotomy can be used for severe deformity.[2] To offer a percutaneous solution to all severities of deformity, a basal closing wedge osteotomy for the severe deformity that cannot be corrected with a distal osteotomy was also developed.

INDICATIONS OR CONTRAINDICATIONS

The chevron and the basal closing wedge osteotomy are established techniques to correct mild to moderate reducible[3–5] severe deformity. The authors consider that a severe deformity, with an IMA greater than 20°, is not necessarily a contraindication for a percutaneous chevron osteotomy. The procedure selection depends on the relationship between the width of the head and the first or second intermetatarsal distance. If there is a modification of the distal metatarsal articular angle (DMAA), a distal chevron is preferred.[4] Individuals factors, such as the quality of the bone and the age of the patient, should be discussed. If both the chevron and the basal osteotomy are possible, the choice depends on the possibility of the patient bearing weight on the heel during the 6 weeks following the surgery. If necessary, a combined procedure (chevron plus basal osteotomy) can be performed. The main contraindications are active infection and critical arterial occlusive disease.

SURGICAL TECHNIQUE

The preoperative planning includes a full history of the pathologic condition, a clinical examination, and a radiologic assessment. The severity of the deformity is measured by the mobility of the first metatarsophalangeal (MTP) and tarsometatarsal (TMT) joints, the presence of a callus, and the reducibility of the deformity. Association of lesser ray deformity and consequences on the patient's activities and footwear are noted. The maximal IMA is evaluated by squeezing the first space with 1 or 2 fingers (squeeze test) (**Fig. 1**). The size of the head is clinically appreciated. The radiographic evaluation (standing AP and lateral views) is carried out considering the IMA, hallux valgus angle, proximal phalangeal articular angle, DMAA measurements, lateral

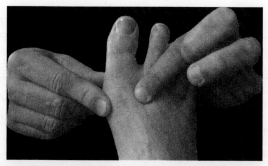

Fig. 1. The squeeze test. The first metatarsal interspace is pressed with 1 or 2 fingers to evaluate the maximal IMA. The index finger and the thumb pinch the first space at the level of the head and, if possible, the middle finger is placed against the index finger.

subluxation of the sesamoids, and the width of the head compared with the width of the first intermetatarsal web space. The choice of the procedure between a distal chevron (MICA) and a basal is then made.

The preparation and patient positioning are the same for the both techniques. The procedure is performed under general anesthesia and/or ankle block. The advantage of an isolated ankle block is the exclusive sensitive action, which allows the patient to partially weight bear after the surgery. No tourniquet is required. The foot is placed over the end of the table to allow intraoperative radiographs to be easily obtained. The authors recommend the use of a mini C-arm (**Fig. 2**).

The surgical approach requires a Beaver blade Beaver®, a Shannon burr with a length of 20 mm × 2 mm wide or 12 mm × 2 mm, and a wedge burr with a length of 13 mm × 3.1 mm wide. A specific driver system with high torque and low speed is required. This offers a good ratio between cutting the bone and the risk of burning the skin. A speed of less than 10,000 rpm is recommended.

The Surgical Procedure

The percutaneous chevron osteotomy with extreme displacement (MICA) technique is similar to the percutaneous chevron for mild to moderate deformity. The difference is in the translation and the fixation (**Fig. 3**):

1. The osteotomy is performed with a Shannon burr of 20 mm × 2 mm at the flare of the neck of the metatarsal and is extra-articular. The plane of the apex of the chevron is controlled under an image intensifier. To obtain a neutral translation in consideration of length or elevation, the burr must be oriented perpendicular to the first metatarsal with a plantar angle of 10° (**Fig. 4**). When the direction of the apex is correct, the dorsal and plantar cuts are created.
2. After performing the osteotomy and before the translation, the fixation is prepared. It is a 2-screw fixation from medial to lateral. The proximal screw must be bicortical in the metatarsal before penetrating the head. The second, parallel to the proximal one, does not need to be systematically bicortical. We use cannulated screws. The proximal K-wire is inserted at the base of the metatarsal with a direction to end up 1 cm lateral to the metatarsal head, penetrating the lateral cortex at a reasonable

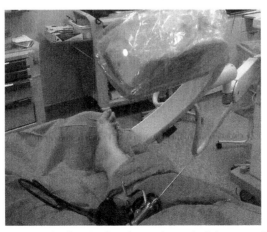

Fig. 2. Patient positioning. The foot is placed over the end of the operating table. The mini C-arm is positioned on the right side of the table if the surgeon is right-handed.

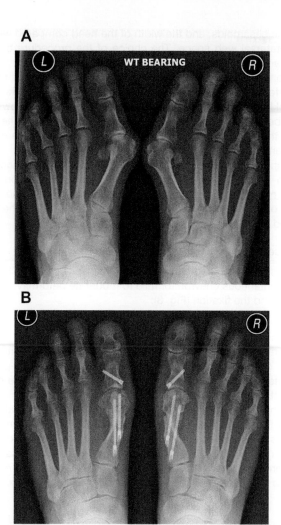

Fig. 3. The MICA. A percutaneous chevron osteotomy with an extreme displacement. (*A*) Preoperative weight (WT) bearing radiograph. (*B*) Postoperative weight bearing radiograph at 4 months after a bilateral correction.

distance of the osteotomy. The entry point is one-third dorsal and two-thirds plantar because of the proximal shape of the metatarsal. The K-wire is aimed toward the osteotomy portal, with a lateral direction to the second MTP joint (**Fig. 5**).
3. The translation is then performed with a specific lever to displace the head up to 100% laterally, if necessary (**Fig. 6**). The medial metatarsal wall can be fractured in the elderly patient by the levering instrument. Applying a varus of the first phalanx is necessary to avoid an associated rotation of the head.
4. Once the correction is obtained with the desired displacement, the K-wire is pushed into the head. The wire is measured and a screw is inserted (a diameter of 4 mm is recommended for large displacement). A second screw of 3 mm is then inserted parallel to the first screw. It is important to check the position of the screw in AP and lateral views. A flanged head screw is used to obtain a strong fixation with a nonprominent screw head (**Fig. 7**).

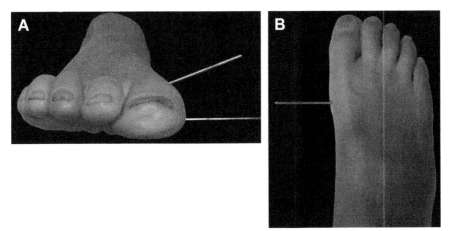

Fig. 4. The plane of the apex of the chevron. (*A*) The orientation of the apex dictates the final displacement of the head. (*B*) A neutral translation is obtained with an apex perpendicular to the first metatarsal and an angle of 10° dorsal from plantar.

5. The medial wall of the metatarsal becomes redundant and needs to be removed with a burr inserted from the distal screw or osteotomy portal (**Fig. 8**).
6. Percutaneous distal soft-tissue release is performed if necessary, if the correction needs it and must be performed after the translation and fixation of the osteotomy.

The percutaneous basal closing wedge osteotomy technique is based on the standard closing wedge osteotomy described for an open procedure (**Fig. 9**). The procedure is controlled under an image intensifier:

1. The M1M2 angle must be manually increased to maximum and temporally fixed in position. We use a 2 mm K-wire inserted at the base of the metatarsal, parallel to

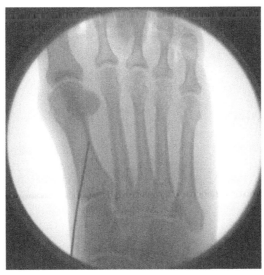

Fig. 5. The fixation, first stage. The fixation is planned before the displacement by positioning the K-wire for the cannulated screw proximally in the first metatarsal from the medial to the lateral cortex.

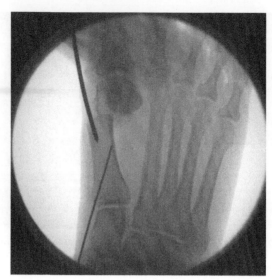

Fig. 6. The fixation, second stage. The translation is obtained with a lever introduced through the osteotomy approach intramedullary in the metatarsal diaphysis.

the TMT joint, and pinned into the second metatarsal. Simultaneously, a dorsal flexion of the first metatarsal is applied at the level of the TMT joint (**Fig. 10**).

2. The osteotomy is performed with a Shannon burr of 20 mm × 2 mm from a 3 mm dorsal proximal portal. The burr is introduced in the middle of the bone, lateral to the extensor, to avoid any nerve damage, from dorsal to plantar. The osteotomy starts from medial proximal to lateral distal, with the preservation of the upper medial cortex. It is important to keep the medial dorsal cortex intact to prevent elevation of the metatarsal (**Fig. 11**).

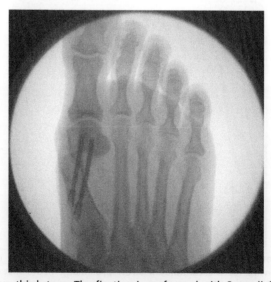

Fig. 7. The fixation, third stage. The fixation is performed with 2 parallel screws.

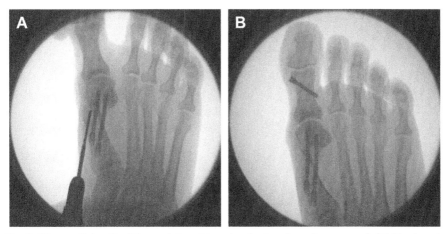

Fig. 8. The medial wall of the metatarsal is redundant and can be removed. (*A*) The burr is introduced under the medial wall. (*B*) The medial wall is removed.

3. The osteotomy is closed and the correction is evaluated. At this stage, the wedge is not wide enough to correct the deformity.
4. A 3.1 mm wedge burr is then introduced in the osteotomy to widen the wedge until a complete correction is obtained (**Fig. 12**). The reaming will preserve the lateral wall. The control of the correction is frequent to avoid any excess.

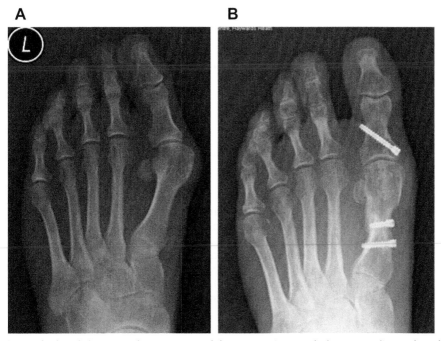

Fig. 9. The basal closing wedge osteotomy. (*A*) Preoperative weight bearing radiograph and (*B*) postoperative weight bearing radiograph at 3 months.

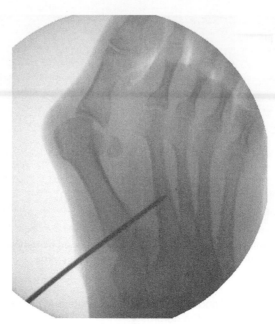

Fig. 10. Temporary fixation of the first metatarsal with a K-wire between M1 and M2 in a maximal IMA and a dorsal flexion of the TMT.

5. The osteotomy is then closed manually and the fixation is realized with 2 screws of 3 mm from medial to lateral inserted over a temporary 1 mm K-wire. The positions are controlled with an image intensifier (**Fig. 13**).
6. Percutaneous distal soft-tissue release is performed if necessary, if the correction needs it and it can be performed before the osteotomy.
7. The decision to perform an Akin osteotomy depends on the remaining deformity at the level of the interphalangeal angle. The surgery requires a Shannon burr of 12 mm × 2 mm via a midaxial medial portal. The burr is introduced in the phalanx from distal to proximal. The osteotomy preserves the lateral cortex. The osteotomy is closed in varus. The fixation is performed with a screw proximal to distal and medial to lateral (**Fig. 14**).
8. Suture of the skin portal is not required; it can be closed with Steri-Strips (Elastoplast ®). Wet gauze is applied. The dressing is completed with Elastoplast, or wool and crepe bandages (**Fig. 15**).

Complications and Management

The potential list of complications is the same as for the open procedure. The main risks and pitfalls are connected to the position of the portal, the position of the osteotomy, and the quality of the fixation. That is why it is mandatory that the surgeon who chooses to perform this procedure has cadaveric training to avoid such complications, particularly for the chevron osteotomy and the positioning of the proximal K-wire. If it is too close to the osteotomy, the cortical may break when the screw is inserted or, secondarily, when the patient begins weight bearing.

Postoperative Care

Postoperative care depends on the procedure. A distal chevron osteotomy allows full weight bearing in an orthopedic flat shoe, whereas a basal closing wedge will require

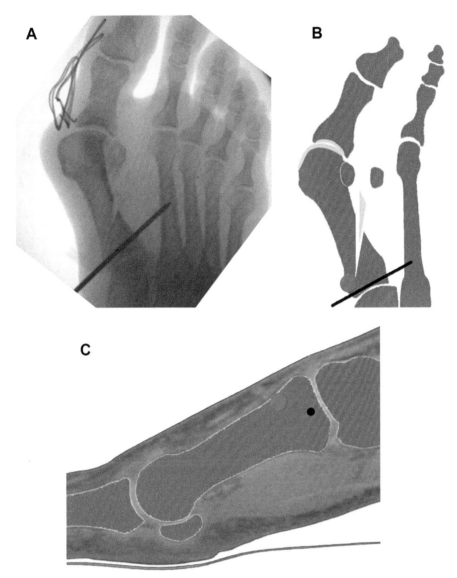

Fig. 11. The osteotomy, first stage. This is performed with a Shannon burr 20 mm × 2 mm and must preserve the dorsal and medial corner (*Red dot*). (*A*) Preoperative radiograph, (*B*) axial view of the medial dorsal corner, and (*C*) lateral view of the medial dorsal corner.

an orthopedic heel-bearing shoe. Deep vein thrombosis (DVT) prophylaxis is not typical. Chemoprophylaxis may be prescribed if there is history of previous DVT (**Table 1**).

Outcomes

There are few published data of results for both techniques; however, both show excellent results in terms of correction and satisfaction (**Table 2**).

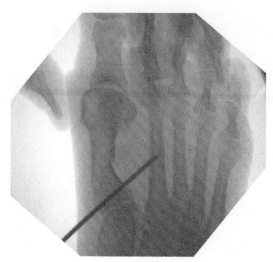

Fig. 12. The osteotomy, second stage. A wedge burr 3.1 mm is necessary to increase the wedge to obtain the perfect correction.

The authors noticed more stiffness with the basal osteotomy than the MICA but this was not reflected with the different scores.

Summary

The correction of a severe hallux valgus deformity is a great challenge. It starts with the proper evaluation of the deformity. Although the full weight bearing radiographs are useful, they do not perfectly assess the potential deformity and deformation during the gait. Frequently, the full weight bearing radiograph undervalues the real instability at the level of the TMT joint. That is why a clinical test such as the squeeze test is particularly valuable. The purpose is to evaluate the true potential IMA. The first space is pressed between the index finger and the thumb at the level of the head and, if

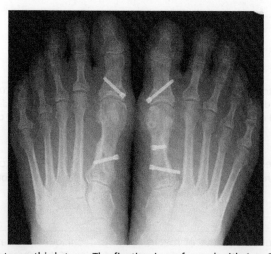

Fig. 13. The osteotomy, third stage. The fixation is performed with 1 or 2 screws.

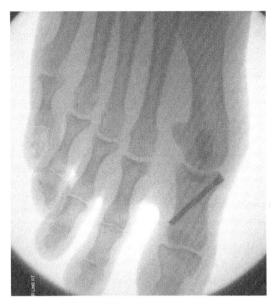

Fig. 14. The akin osteotomy is fixed with a screw.

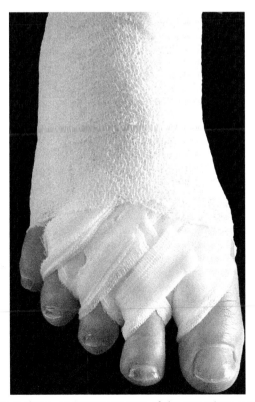

Fig. 15. The dressing is always an important part of the procedure, particularly if an additional procedure on the lesser ray has been performed.

Table 1 Minimally invasive chevron and Akin compared with basal closing wedge postoperative care		
	MICA	Basal Closing Wedge
Foot elevate 45 min/h	Yes	Yes
Calf exercise	Yes	Yes
Compression stocking	Contralateral	Contralateral
DVT prophylaxis	Not systematic	Not systematic
Orthopedic shoe	Flat	Heel
Orthopedic shoe	4–5 wk	6 wk
Weight bearing	Full	Heel (partial)
Dressing	2 wk	2 wk
Follow-up	2–6 wk & 3 mo	2–6 wk & 3 mo
Review	1 y	1 y

possible, the middle finger is placed against the index finger. This maneuver is reproduced at the beginning of the surgery to confirm the deformity. With this maneuver, the mobility of the TMT is evaluated. This allows the surgeon to determine the required displacement to correct the deformity the surgeon must place the head of the metatarsal on the top of the sesamoid. The size of the first metatarsal head must be clinically and radiologically appreciated. On the full weight bearing radiograph with the measurement of the hallux valgus and the IMA, the surgeon may measure the distance between the lateral cortex of the first metatarsal head to the medial cortex of the second metatarsal head (a) and the width of the first metatarsal head (b). It is the ratio between these 2 measurements that determines the choice of the procedure (interspace ratio = a/b). If the ratio is less than or equal to 1, then an MICA is used to achieve the correction of the deformity. With a result equal to 1, the displacement is 100% of the diameter of the head. If the ratio is greater than 1, a proximal closing wedge is the chosen procedure (**Fig. 16**).

The age of the patient, the quality of the bone, and the implications of each procedure must be taken into account. If the basal osteotomy is used to correct the deformity, heel weight bearing is required for 6 weeks. This condition can be difficult or impossible for a disabled or elderly patient. Few techniques have been described for severe hallux valgus deformity. None were reported using a percutaneous technique until recently by De Lavigne and colleagues.[6] The authors prefer basal closing wedge technique. A basal osteotomy, because it is a rotation, closes the M1M2 angle. However, it paradoxically lengthens the first ray. Indeed, the cosine of a small angle is higher than the cosine of a large one. This is responsible for a temporary stiffness at the level of the first MTP joint. The open closing wedge has been abandoned for a medial open wedge osteotomy. The open wedge offers the comfort of a simple, easy to fix approach. However, performing an open wedge osteotomy, even if it is simpler, increases the length of the first ray. The stiffness is secondary to the tension of the soft tissue and tendon. Because it is a rotation, it can increase the distal metatarsal articular angle and needs an additional distal osteotomy to correct it. A proximal osteotomy, if it is more powerful, can potentially have more risk of transfer metatarsalgia.[7] A mistake of 1° of dorsal flexion of a 4 cm metatarsal length could cause an elevation of 0.7 mm of the first metatarsal. That is why it is essential to control the perfect position of the osteotomy by keeping the proximal, dorsal, and medial cortex intact. By preserving it, the closure of the osteotomy is associated to a plantar flexion of the metatarsal.

Table 2
Minimally invasive chevron and Akin compared with basal closing wedge radiographic results

		Hallux Valgus		IMA			
		Preoperative	Postoperative	Preoperative	Postoperative	Complications	Satisfaction
Basal closing wedge	J. Vernois	35.4°	12.6°	14.8°	6.6°	1/100	98%
Percutaneous double metatarsal osteotomy[6]	C. De Lavigne	43°	16°	22°	11°	0	—
Percutaneous chevron[2]	J. Vernois	33.7°	7.3°	14.5°	5.5°	7/341	95%

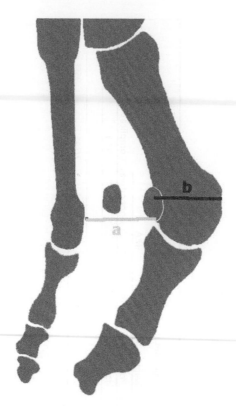

Fig. 16. How to evaluate the potential distal correction. a, distance between the lateral border of the hallux head and the medial border of the second metatarsal; b, width of the hallux head.

With the MICA, a displacement of 100% is possible due to the quality of the fixation. Although it can be used easily in most patients and deformities, the result of a nearly normal foot is better with a basal osteotomy. This is an aesthetic aspect that is valued nowadays. The potential osteonecrosis of the head has not been reported with this technique,[8] probably because the osteotomy is extra-articular more proximally.

Both techniques show excellent results. Their indications can be stackable in terms of deformity but the choice depends on different considerations (**Table 3**).

Table 3
Minimally invasive chevron and Akin compared with basal closing wedge indications

	MICA	Basal Closing Wedge
Interspace ratio ≤1	Yes	Yes
Interspace ratio >1	No	Yes
DMAA normal	Yes	Yes
DMAA pathologic	Yes	No or double osteotomy
Metatarsalgia	Yes	Yes
Disabled patient	Yes	No
Quality bone poor	Yes	No

SUMMARY

Severe hallux valgus is a challenge to treat. Chevron and basal osteotomy percutaneous procedures have been recently described. A basal osteotomy is a well-known surgery for severe deformity and the chevron osteotomy is often used for mild to moderate deformity. The evolution of this fixation (MICA) allows it to be used with severe deformity. With a maximum displacement of 100%, the MICA offers a reliable technique for all deformities. The limit of the technique is a severe IMA with a small head. A percutaneous basal closing wedge osteotomy is used to correct such a deformity. Percutaneous techniques are adequate procedures to correct all deformities. Surgeons need appropriate cadaveric training to gain the appropriate experience.

REFERENCES

1. Vernois J, Jarde O, Havet E, et al. Résultat d'une série préliminaire de chevron percutané dans le traitement de l'hallux valgus. Assoc Fançaise Chir Pied Résumés Journ AFCP 2007. Available at: http://www.afcp.com.fr/. Accessed November 20, 2008.
2. Vernois J, David Redfern, Grecmip. Percutaneous Chevron; the union of classic stable fixed approach and percutaneous technique. Fuß & Sprunggelenk 2013; 11(2):70–5.
3. Austin DW, Leventen EO. A new osteotomy for hallux valgus: a horizontally directed "V" displacement osteotomy of the metatarsal head for hallux valgus and primus varus. Clin Orthop Relat Res 1981;(157):25–30.
4. Nery C, Barroco R, Réssio C. Biplanar chevron osteotomy. Foot Ankle Int 2002; 23(9):792–8.
5. Trnka HJ, Zembsch A, Wiesauer H, et al. Modified Austin procedure for correction of hallux valgus. Foot Ankle Int 1997;18(3):119–27.
6. De Lavigne C, Rasmont Q, Hoang B. Percutaneous double metatarsal osteotomy for correction of severe hallux valgus deformity. Acta Orthop Belg 2011;77(4): 516–21.
7. García-Bordes I, Jiménez-Potrero M, Voga García J, et al. Opening first metatarsal osteotomy and resection arthroplasty of the first MPJ in the treatment of first ray insufficiency associated with degenerative hallux valgus. Foot Ankle Surg 2010;16(3):132–6.
8. Meier PJ, Kenzora JE. The risks and benefits of distal first metatarsal osteotomies. Foot Ankle 1985;6(1):7–17.

Managing Complications of Percutaneous Surgery of the First Metatarsal

Shu-Yuan Li, MD, PhD[a], Jian-Zhong Zhang, MD[a],*,
Yong-Tao Zhang, MS[b]

KEYWORDS

- Percutaneous osteotomy • Minimal invasive surgery • Hallux valgus • Complication
- Revision

KEY POINTS

- The percutaneous osteotomy technique, as a treatment option for hallux valgus, has had a high popularity for both patients and surgeons over the past 2 decades in the mainland of China.
- The procedure is performed similarly to what was done in the United States in the 1970s with a linear distal first metatarsal osteotomy but with no fixation.
- Complications of percutaneous surgery of the first metatarsal can generally be predictably corrected with arthrodesis of the first metatarsophalangeal joint.
- In order to provide a stable medial column, arthrodesis should be the best treatment of choice in cases where substantial bone has been lost.

 Video content accompanies this article at http://www.foot.theclinics.com.

INTRODUCTION

Hallux valgus is a common forefoot deformity, with adduction of the first metatarsal and valgus deviation of the first metatarsophalangeal joint (MTP). The primary complaints are prominence and discomfort of the bunion, limitation in range of motion of the MTP joint, and associated or subsequent lesser toe problems, such as hammer toe, cross-over toe, metatarsalgia. Treatments include conservative management and surgeries. However, effects of conservative treatment, such as shoes

Disclosure Statement: The authors have nothing to disclose.
[a] Foot and Ankle Center, Orthopaedic Department, Beijing Tongren Hospital, Capital Medical University, No. 1 Dongjiaominxiang Street, Dongcheng District, Beijing 100730, China;
[b] Orthopedics and Traumatology Department, Zibo Combinational Hospital of Chinese and Western Medicine, No 8. Jinjing Street, Zhangdian District, Zibo City, Shandong Province 255026, China
* Corresponding author.
E-mail address: trfoot@126.com

modification, using orthotics or insoles, are not so promising and definite, and many patients have to resort to surgery when conservative managements do not work.

Although there are more than one hundred types of surgeries described for the correction of hallux valgus deformity, the goals for treatment remain the same, that is, to realign the first ray, maintain or maximize the range of motion of the MTP joint, and to treat the related deformities of the forefoot. Percutaneous surgery on the forefoot was described by Morton Polokoff[1] in 1945 using fine instruments such as chisels, rasps, and spears. Later Leonard Britton[1] tried to treat hallux valgus deformities with percutaneous first metatarsal opening, closing, and dorsiflexion wedge osteotomies as well as Akin osteotomy. However, it was in the 1970s when minimally invasive surgery of the foot was developed by North American podiatrists.[1,2] With the introduction of minimum incision and percutaneous procedures into the curriculum at Pennsylvania College of Podiatric Medicine in 1974,[3] and low-intensity radiographic imaging scope into the practice,[4] this kind of technique, based on a Hohmann-type metatarsal subcapital linear osteotomy,[5] rapidly became popular. At that time, no internal fixation was used for stabilization of the osteotomy. In the 1980s, Peter Bösch combined this percutaneous osteotomy with an internal axial Steinmann pin fixation technique as described by Lamprecht and Kramer and named this new technique "subcutaneous Bösch technique."[6–8] Most of present percutaneous procedures are modifications of the Bösch technique.

The percutaneous osteotomy technique was introduced into Mainland China in the late 1980s. In the following 20 years, there has been little development or modification, so the surgical procedure being used nowadays in Mainland China is still similar to what was commonly used among the podiatrists in United States in the 1970s, which consists of a linear distal first metatarsal osteotomy through a medial approach, with soft tissue release on the lateral side of the first MTP being rarely used. The osteotomy is performed with a power burr, by perforating the subcapital cortex of the metatarsal, manually breaking, and shifting the distal fragment laterally, with plantar flexing or laterally rotating the metatarsal head according to the actual condition. At the completion of the surgery, the alignment is verified under fluoroscopy; then a compression bandage is used to stabilize the osteotomy and maintain the correction without K-wire fixation.[9] After the surgery, immediate ambulation is allowed with forefoot non-weight-bearing shoes or stiff-soled shoes. The special compression bandages are removed at 6 weeks, and patients are allowed to change into normal shoes after radiographic union is confirmed. This type of preparation of the osteotomy without fixation is similar to other forefoot osteotomies described in the twentieth century, including the Ludloff osteotomy, the Hohmann osteotomy, the Helal osteotomy, and others. All of these osteotomies were demonstrated to have a high incidence of complications and were abandoned in that form. Unfortunately, at present in China, there is still a large group of surgeons who continue to perform the procedure without fixation, and the consequences are unpredictable. There are many complications, such as malunion, shortening, nonunion, and others. It is these complications specifically that the authors discuss in this article.

As an alternative method to more traditional open surgeries, the percutaneous technique has achieved rapid acceptance and popularity by patients and surgeons alike over the past 2 decades. Percutaneous forefoot procedures and minimally invasive surgeries for hallux valgus occupy almost 30% of forefoot surgical cases in China today. The high popularity and acceptance by patients in China are due to their general desire for an improved cosmetic outcome and the perceived minimal invasiveness of the surgery and is magnified by the surgeons' efforts to popularize the advantages of this technique over traditional open surgeries, including shorter surgical time, less exposure and soft tissue dissection, faster healing, earlier ambulation, and quicker rehabilitation.

However, despite its high acceptance by patients and high enthusiasm by surgeons at present, the clinical outcomes of percutaneous surgery in the management of hallux valgus in China have not been promising. As the earliest established foot and ankle surgeon team in China, the authors have revised many complications following these percutaneous first metatarsal osteotomies in the past 10 years, although they have never performed any percutaneous osteotomies in their center. The main problems are insufficient correction, first metatarsal shortening, transfer metatarsalgia, elevation of first metatarsal head, first MTP joint incongruence, first MTP joint stiffness, first MTP joint arthritis, hammer toe deformity of lesser toes, delayed union or nonunion of the osteotomy, and avascular necrosis of the first metatarsal head. Revision surgeries were always difficult to perform. Here, some typical cases of poor results of attempted percutaneous first metatarsal osteotomy surgery of the hallux valgus are presented, in order to provide readers with common complications of this technique and options for revision.

TYPICAL CASES
Case 1

A 32-year-old woman presented to the authors with stiff dysfunctional great toes on both sides and very painful calluses under bilateral second metatarsal heads. The patient received bilateral percutaneous osteotomy of the first metatarsal in another hospital 2 years before (**Fig. 1**). Physical examination showed that the 2 great toes were all short with stiff first MTP joints. The right great toe was in a slight varus. On both sides, the medial column was lifted with less weight-bearing than normal. The second toe on both sides had a hammer toe deformity, with a slight dorsal subluxation on the sagittal plane, and lateral deviation on the horizontal plane. There was a large callus underneath the second metatarsal head of both sides, with significant tenderness (**Figs. 2 and 3**). The diagnosis was transfer metatarsalgia caused by shortening and elevation of the first metatarsal. Treatment could be conservative with padding and orthotic support or various types of surgical procedures designed to improve the first ray function by lengthening and plantarflexing the first metatarsal, and shortening the second metatarsal to get a balanced forefoot load distribution. The patient was reluctant to

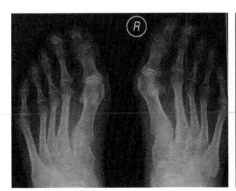
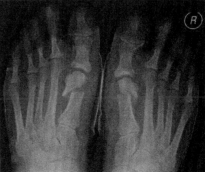

Fig. 1. (*Left*) Preoperative AP view. Hallux valgus present; note the relative lengths of the first and second metatarsal. (*Right*) Immediate postoperative AP view. Note the shortening of the first metatarsal and the slight varus deformity of the hallux toes.

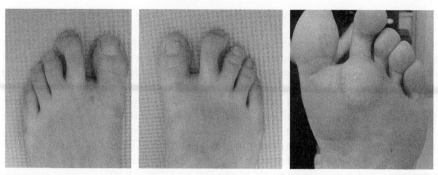

Fig. 2. Subsequent postoperative views of the dorsal and plantar surfaces. Note the excessively short hallux toes (*left and middle*) and the callosity under the second metatarsal head (*right*). There is also deformity with lateral deviation of the second toe indicative of overload.

have surgery, and orthotic treatment was used to balance the forefoot load distribution with improvement of the metatarsalgia.

Case 2

A 54-year-old female patient presented to the authors' clinic with a painful and deformed second toe on her left foot, 4 years after a percutaneous surgery for correcting hallux valgus. Physical examination demonstrated that the second toe was a fixed hammer toe deformity with a dorsally dislocated MTP joint and a stiff irreducible proximal interphalangeal (PIP) joint. Painful callus was found both on the dorsum of the PIP joint and underneath the metatarsal head of the second toe. The short great toe had a good range of motion and no pain during weight-bearing or in movement. There was no elevation of the first metatarsal (**Fig. 4**). Radiographic examination showed a shortened first metatarsal, and a dorsally dislocated second MTP joint (**Fig. 5**). Diagnosis for this patient was still transfer metatarsalgia caused by excessive shortening of the first metatarsal.

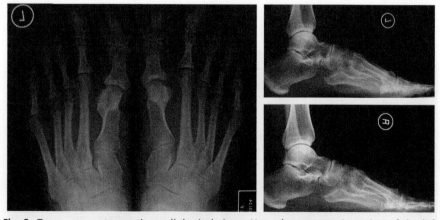

Fig. 3. Two-years postoperative radiological views. Note the severe orientation of the left foot with hallux varus and the marked shortening of the first metatarsal (*left*). Note that the bilateral first metatarsals are not only short but also elevated at the metatarsal neck, further aggravating the second metatarsal overload (*right upper and lower*).

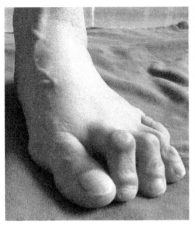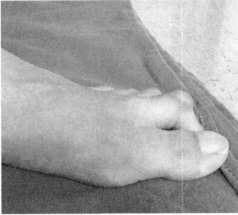

Fig. 4. Four-years postoperative views of the dorsal and lateral surfaces. Note the hammer toe deformities in the lateral toes, especially the second toe, with callosity on the dorsum of the PIP joint.

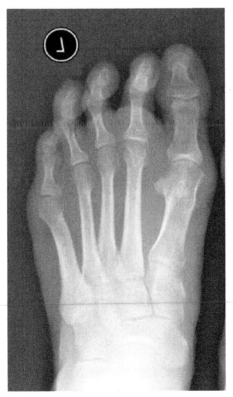

Fig. 5. Four-years postoperative radiological photograph. Note the marked shortening of the first metatarsal, and dorsal dislocation of the second MTP joint.

For this case, the authors chose to treat the symptomatic second toe first. After shortening the second metatarsal with a modified Weil osteotomy, the dislocated MTP joint reduced, and the length discrepancy between I first and second was gone. The fixed PIP joint of the second toe was fixed with arthroplasty and a K-wire. Because the great toe functioned well, no surgical procedure was done on the first metatarsal. After shortening the second metatarsal, the third metatarsal head got relatively prominent, and a slight shortening of the third metatarsal with a modified Weil osteotomy was performed to improve the transfer metatarsalgia on the third toe (**Fig. 6**). Two-year postoperative follow-up visit demonstrated that the patient was doing well without further transfer metatarsalgia to the fourth.

Case 3

A 53-year-old female patient presented to the authors with severe bilateral forefoot pain in weight-bearing 5 years after percutaneous surgery. Complications were similar to case 2, which were caused by shortening of the first metatarsal bilaterally (**Fig. 7**). However, in this case, there was arthritis of the first MTP joints as well as dislocation of second and third MTP joints (**Fig. 8**). The authors had the option of performing an in situ arthrodesis of the hallux MTP joint, particularly because the lesser metatarsals were going to be substantially shortened through the osteotomies. The in situ arthrodesis of the MTP joint is far easier to perform than the bone block graft, but the patient

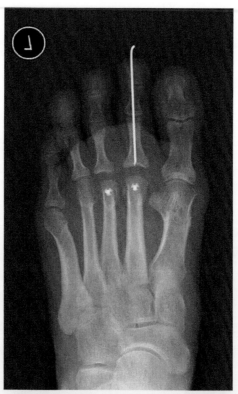

Fig. 6. Immediate AP view after revision surgery. Note after shortening of the second and third metatarsals, and the arthroplasty procedure performed on the PIP joint of the second toe, length of first to third metatarsals was balanced.

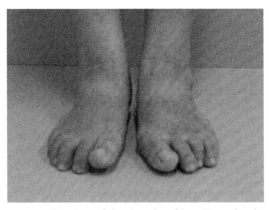

Fig. 7. Five-years postoperative view of the dorsal surfaces. Note the shortening and elevation of the bilateral great toes, and hammer toe deformity of the lateral toes.

desired maximum cosmesis as well as function. Therefore, the first MTP joint arthrodesis was performed with a structural iliac crest autograft block bone graft, and modified Weil osteotomies on the second to fourth metatarsals were performed, with fusion of PIP joint of the second toe to treat the irreducible hammer toe (see **Fig. 8**).

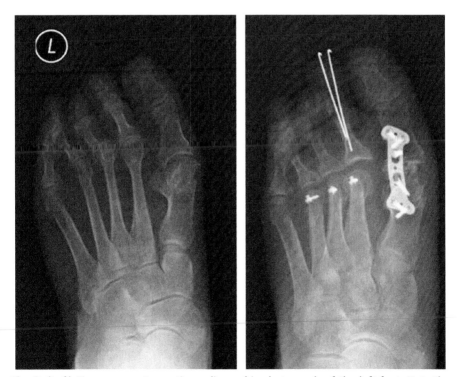

Fig. 8. (*Left*) Five-years postoperative radiographic photograph of the left foot. Note the marked shortening of the first metatarsal, arthritis in first MTP joint, as well as dislocation of second and third MTP joints. (*Right*) Immediate AP view after revision surgery. Note the first MTP joint arthrodesis with a structural bone block graft, and the shortening of the second to fourth metatarsals with modified Weil osteotomies, and fusion of PIP joint of the second toe.

Case 4

A 75-year-old woman came to the authors' clinic with intolerable pain under bilateral forefeet in weight-bearing. She had bilateral percutaneous surgeries on the great toe 4 years before. Both of her great toes were very short, and slightly floppy in elevation, and not bearing any load. There were also diffuse calluses under lesser metatarsals as a sign of overloading (**Fig. 9**). Gastrocnemius muscles on both sides were tight. Radiological examination revealed that the bilateral first metatarsals were very short, and the first MTP joints were incongruent and unstable with a narrow joint space (**Fig. 10**). Based on this, the diagnosis was bilateral shortening of the first metatarsal, first MTP joint arthritis, and transfer metatarsalgia of lesser toes.

For this case, what kind of surgical plan should be used, lengthening the first metatarsal, or shortening the lateral lesser metatarsals, or both? In consideration of the patient's older age, degeneration of bilateral first MTP joints, and great length discrepancy between the first metatarsal and the lesser ones, the authors decided to combine the above described procedures together, that is, lengthening and stabilizing the first column with MTP joint arthrodesis and shortening the lateral second to fourth metatarsals with modified Weil osteotomy. Once again as with the previous case, the authors had the option of an in situ arthrodesis or a lengthening arthrodesis of the hallux MTP joint. This decision was difficult in a patient of this age, because the extent of the procedure and the length of time to incorporate the graft are considerably greater. The recovery process is different as well, because the patient is not allowed to bear weight for an extended period of time. One has to understand the mechanical structure of the forefoot with an arthrodesis of the MTP joint performed in a shortened position in conjunction with shortening of the lesser metatarsals. The authors see and treat this condition frequently in patients with rheumatoid arthritis, under very similar circumstances. An in situ arthrodesis is performed, often with shortening of the metatarsal, in conjunction with resection of the lesser metatarsal heads. These patients function very well, and similarly in this patient, the authors had to decide if an in situ arthrodesis would be sufficient and thought that due to the excessive shortening that lengthening with a structural graft would be advantageous. Structural bone grafts were used in the MTP joints arthrodesis. Because there was symptomatic fifth toe varus bilaterally, bilateral chevron osteotomies were performed and fixed with K-wires

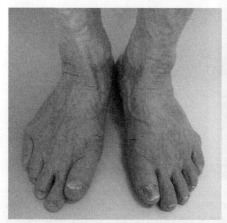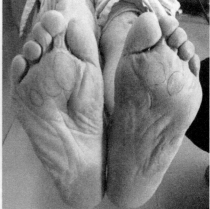

Fig. 9. Four-years postoperative view of the dorsal and plantar surfaces. Note obvious shortening and elevation of the bilateral great toes, and diffuse calluses under lesser metatarsals.

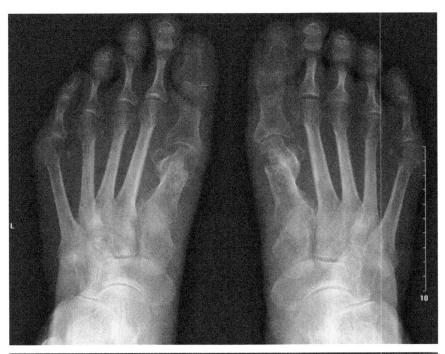

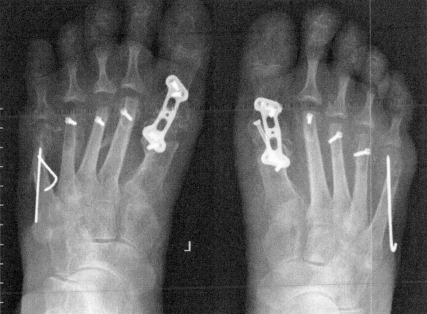

Fig. 10. (*Upper row*) Four-years postoperative radiological photograph of bilateral feet. Note the shortened first metatarsals and the incongruent first MTP joints. (*Lower row*) Immediate AP view after the revision surgery. Note the first MTP joint arthrodesis with structural bone block graft, and the shortening of the second to fourth metatarsals with modified Weil osteotomies, and correction of fifth varus toe with chevron osteotomies bilaterally.

(see **Fig. 10**). A gastrocnemius release procedure was also performed to help relieve the loading of the forefeet.

Case 5

A 50-year-old female patient who underwent bilateral percutaneous osteotomy surgeries 4 years previously presented to the authors. She developed continuous unimproved pain underneath both of her forefeet, with the second and third toes becoming gradually deformed. The patient came to the authors' clinic for a revision surgery of her left foot, which had more severe symptoms than the right foot. Physical examination showed obvious shortening and pronation deformity of the bilateral great toes and hammer toe deformity of the lateral second and third toes. The PIP joints of bilateral second toes were stiff and irreducible. There were diffuse calluses under lesser metatarsals, indicating overloading (**Fig. 11**). Radiological examination showed significant shortening of bilateral first metatarsals, incongruent first MTP joints with excessive bunionectomy, and residual untreated large distal metatarsal articular angle (DMAA). The intermetatarsal angle (IMA) and hallux valgus angle (HVA) were all large because of insufficient correction or recurrence of the previous percutaneous surgery. On lateral view, elevation of the first metatarsal and dorsal subluxation of the second MTP joint were found bilaterally (**Fig. 12**). Based on the above information, the diagnosis was as follows: shortening of first metatarsal, incongruent first MTP joint, irreducible hammer toe of second toe, transfer metatarsalgia.

The principle of treating transfer metatarsalgia is always similar, that is, either lengthening the first metatarsal or shortening the lateral metatarsals, or a combination of both. In this case, besides transfer metatarsalgia and deformities of lesser toes, there was uncorrected hallux valgus deformity as well, with large IMA, HVA, and pronation of the proximal phalanx. Given the multiplanar nature of the deformity, an arthrodesis would be the choice of most surgeons, and this would be a good procedure under the circumstances. An arthrodesis was refused by the patient, and the revision osteotomy needed to have the ability of correcting the hallux valgus, and lengthening and plantar flexing the first metatarsal. For this purpose, a medial side open wedge osteotomy was performed with a custom plate. Because the medial open lengthening could increase the compression on the first MTP joint, it was carefully done by using a plate with a wedge of 8-mm thickness. Modified Weil osteotomies were performed on the second and third metatarsal as well to shorten the metatarsals and reduce the subluxated MTP joints. For correcting the pronation deformity of the hallux, an Akin osteotomy was added (**Fig. 13**).

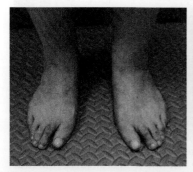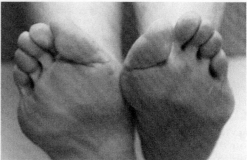

Fig. 11. Four-years postoperative view of the dorsal and plantar surfaces. Note obvious shortening and pronation of the bilateral great toes, hammer toe deformities in second and third toes, and diffuse calluses under bilateral lesser metatarsal heads.

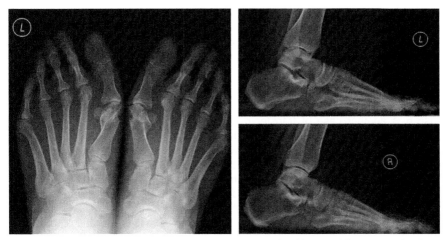

Fig. 12. Four-years postoperative radiological photograph of bilateral feet. Note the shortened first metatarsals, and the incongruent first MTP joints.

However, the surgical treatment of this case still has its drawbacks. It can be found that the first MTP joint was incongruent and unstable with less residual facet on the metatarsal head and a large uncorrected DMAA. As noted above, joint arthrodesis would be the most reliable treatment for this deformity. The last anteroposterior (AP)

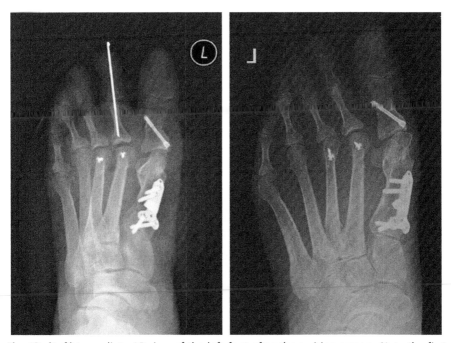

Fig. 13. (*Left*) Immediate AP view of the left foot after the revision surgery. Note the first metatarsal lengthening with medial open osteotomy, and the shortening of the second and third metatarsals with modified Weil osteotomies, and PIP joint fusion of the second toe. (*Right*) One year after the revision surgery. Note the recurrence of the hallux valgus associated with arthritis of the first MTP joint.

view was taken at 1-year follow-up, and although there is recurrence, the hallux valgus, as well as arthritis of the joint (see **Fig. 13**), the treatment was still acceptable to the patient. Because the patient was young, and there was no pain in the first MTP joint before revision surgery, for her age, the opening wedge osteotomy was a better option than joint fusion.

Case 6

Case 6 is another case of transfer metatarsalgia. The patient was a 47-year-old woman, presenting with severe pain under the 2 to 4 metatarsal of her left foot after she received a percutaneous osteotomy surgery for hallux valgus 2 years before (**Fig. 14**). From the preoperative radiological photographs, the authors found that there was a severe shortening of the first metatarsal (**Fig. 15**). The previous surgeon tried to compensate the shortening with intentional plantar displacement of the metatarsal head to avoid transferring the load to lateral metatarsals (see **Fig. 15**). Not only did this not work functionally but also this plantarflexion increases the load on the sesamoids so that even though the lesser metatarsals may be protected, there is usually marked sesamoid pain in addition to the lesser metatarsalgia.

For this case, in order to solve the shortening problem in one stage with osteotomy and internal fixation, the authors decided to combine medial first metatarsal lengthening with lateral metatarsal shortening. The patient unfortunately did not want to undergo many osteotomies, and after careful negotiation with the patient, the authors

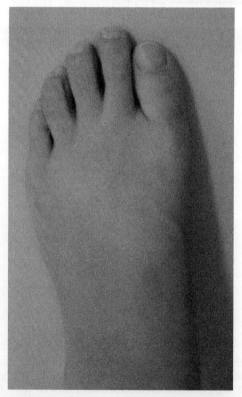

Fig. 14. Two-years postoperative dorsal view of the left foot. Note the excessively short hallux.

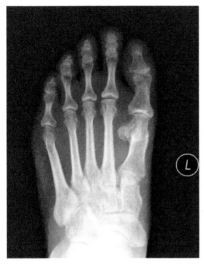

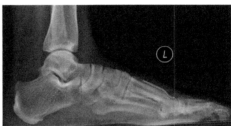

Fig. 15. Two-years postoperative radiological photographs of the left foot. Note the short first metatarsal on the AP view (*left*) and the malunion of the first metatarsal in plantarflexion on the lateral view (*right*). *Red lines* show the outlines of the distal 1st metatarsal, which demonstrates the malunion.

decided to use external fixation for staged lengthening. The staged lengthening was finished in 2.5 months with about 1.5-cm lengthening of the first metatarsal (**Figs. 16** and **17**). Postoperative radiological examination on the 4-month follow-up showed the lengthening result was not acceptable. There was a malunion of the first metatarsal

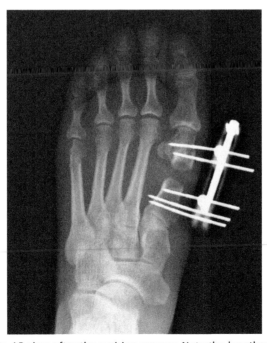

Fig. 16. Immediate AP view after the revision surgery. Note the lengthening procedure of the first metatarsal with external fixation.

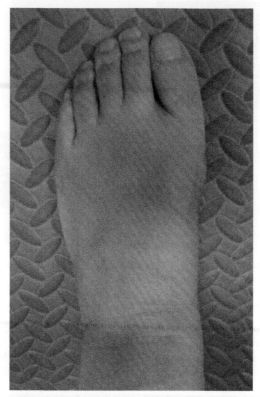

Fig. 17. Four months after the revision surgery. The appearance of the foot was acceptable after the first metatarsal being lengthened.

in plantarflexion (**Fig. 18**); this will lead to increased sesamoid pain, and a dorsal sub-luxation of the hallux MTP joint with dorsal extensor hallux longus (EHL) contracture and lack of function of the hallux.

Case 7

A 28-year-old female patient presented with a stiff and varus big toe and a painful fore-foot on the left side. She had received percutaneous surgical treatment for hallux valgus 2 years previously (**Figs. 19** and **20**). She complained that 6 weeks after the percutaneous surgery, when the compression bandage was removed, her left great toe was found in varus, and there was pain underneath the lateral lesser metatarsals when she was bearing weight. She used orthotics, but there was no significant improvement. She went back to her previous surgeon and received a revision surgery at about 8 months postoperatively. The revision procedure was unclear, but it did not help, and the left great toe was still in varus. She came to us for a revision surgery for both cosmetic and functional reasons.

Physical examination showed the first MTP joint was in varus with movement limi-tation (**Fig. 21**). However, the varus joint could be reduced manually, and after the reduction, a good range of movement was present. There was a significant scar on the dorsal medial side of the joint. Radiological examination demonstrated that there was a negative IMA, which was caused by an aggressive lateral displacement of the distal fragment in the first percutaneous osteotomy, which put the MTP joint in varus

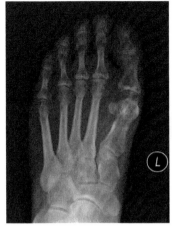
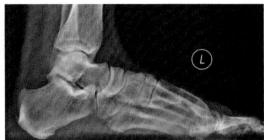

Fig. 18. Radiological photographs of the left foot 4 months after the revision surgery. Note the acceptable length of the first metatarsal on the AP view (*left*) and the worsened malunion of the first metatarsal in plantar flexion on the lateral view (*right*). *Red lines* show the outlines of the distal 1st metatarsal, which demonstrates the malunion.

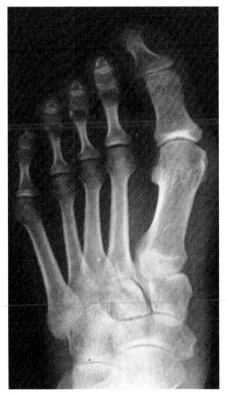

Fig. 19. Preoperative AP view of the left foot. Hallux valgus present; note the relative lengths of the first and second metatarsals.

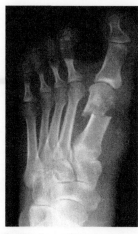
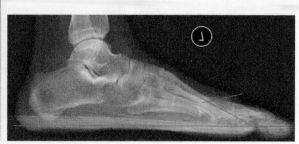

Fig. 20. Immediate postoperative radiological photographs of the left foot. Note the shortening of the first metatarsal after the lateral transverse osteotomy on the AP view (*left*), and the dorsal shift of the first metatarsal head on the lateral view (*right*).

finally. From the lateral view, a dorsal malunion of the osteotomy was found as well, which caused elevation of the first metatarsal head and thus led to transfer metatarsalgia.

In planning the revision surgery, there were concerns as to correction of the hallux varus, with only soft tissue surgery or combining osseous surgery? If osseous surgery

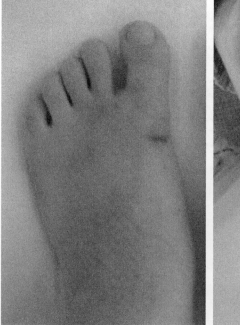
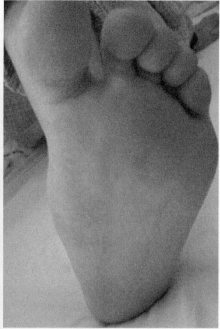

Fig. 21. Two-years postoperative views of the dorsal and plantar surfaces. Note varus and shortening deformity of the great toe and the callosity under the second and third metatarsal heads.

is considered, would it be a joint preservation procedure or not? Besides the dorsal malunion of the first metatarsal head, there was some shortening of the first metatarsal; would it also need to be corrected? After revising the first metatarsal, did the second and third metatarsals need to be shortened to treat the transfer metatarsalgia?

The authors finally chose both soft tissue and osseous procedures to correct the varus deformity. Because the varus first MTP joint could easily be reduced manually, and after reducing the joint, a good range of motion was obtained, the first MTP joint was able to be preserved. The original osteotomy was opened and revised by shifting the distal fragment slight medially and plantarward with structural bone graft being inserted to lengthen the first metatarsal. Then, the osteotomy was fixed with a small low-profile locking plate. However, after lengthening the first metatarsal, the varus deformity of the first MTP joint worsened due to the increased compression from the lengthening across the first MTP joint (**Fig. 22**). To decompress the joint and to correct the deformity, a reverse Akin on lateral side of the proximal phalanx was performed (see **Fig. 22**). After the alignment was checked under fluoroscopy (**Fig. 23**), the extensor hallux brevis tendon was explored, because the authors had planned to use it for correction of the hallux varus. However, they found that it had been damaged during the previous surgeries (**Fig. 24**), and they used a split EHL tendon instead for correction. The tendon was split, and the medial half of the tendon was cut proximally. The proximal end of the tendon was then pulled through the proximal phalangeal base and fixed into a bone tunnel on the medial side cortex of the first metatarsal bone as described originally by Myerson[10] (see **Fig. 24**). The transferred tendon would work as a static structure to reinforce the correction of the hallux varus. Because both the dorsal malunion and shortening of the first metatarsal were corrected, and the forefoot load bearing was redistributed, there was no need to shorten the lateral metatarsals any more (**Fig. 25**).

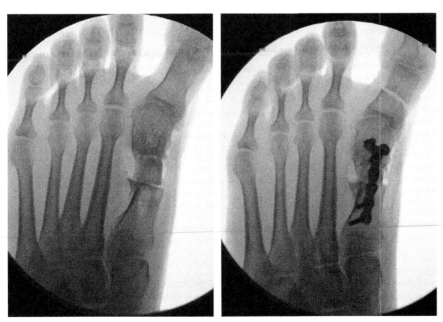

Fig. 22. Intraoperative fluoroscopic AP view during the revision surgery. Note the worsening of the varus deformity after lengthening the first metatarsal with a block bone graft.

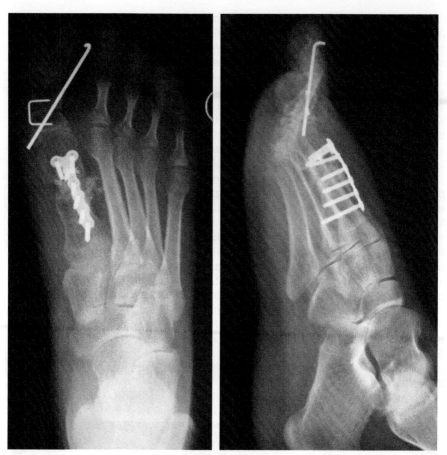

Fig. 23. Intraoperative fluoroscopic AP and lateral views during the revision surgery. Note the correction of the varus deformity with adding a reverse Akin osteotomy on the proximal phalanx of the great toe.

Case 8

A 23-year-old female patient presented with intolerable pain in the interphalangeal (IP) joint under the tip of her left hallux. The patient underwent a percutaneous osteotomy surgery for treating hallux valgus 1 year before. Physical examination demonstrated there was a hammer deformity in the big toe (**Fig. 26**), with severe stiffness of the first MTP joint, hypermobility, and tenderness in the IP joint (Video 1). Radiological examination revealed a large joint facet injury in the MTP joint that was speculated to be caused by the incorrect manipulation during the percutaneous surgery. There was also degenerative arthritis in the IP joint (**Fig. 27**). At this age, this kind of condition is very rare. The IP arthritis was considered to be caused by overloading of the joint due to the stiffness of the MTP joint.

For multiple joint arthritis like this, treatment options are fusion of the first MTP joint and arthroplasty of the PIP joint, or vice versa, arthroplasty of the first MTP and fusion of the PIP joint. However, the patient refused surgeries. Therefore, the authors suggested the patient use conservative treatment with orthotics, nonsteroidal anti-inflammatory drugs, and physical therapy.

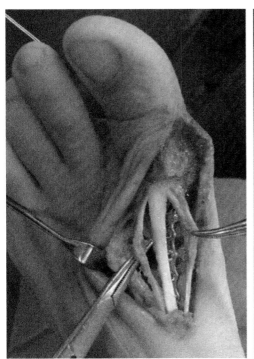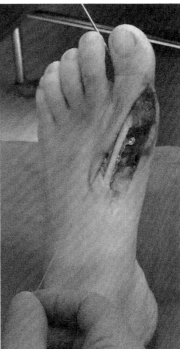

Fig. 24. Intraoperative views of the revision surgery. Note the damaged extensor hallux brevis tendon, and correction of the varus deformity being reinforced by the transferred medial half of the EHL.

DISCUSSION
Percutaneous Osteotomy of the First Metatarsal

For the correction of hallux valgus deformities, more than one hundred correction surgeries have been described in the literature, with different kinds of first metatarsal osteotomies and soft tissue procedures. Among them, no one has been proved to have compelling advantage over the others.[5,6,8,10–14]

Traditionally, osteotomy procedures are performed openly. It can be at the base (proximal osteotomies), on the shaft, or on the head of the first metatarsal (distal osteotomies). Compared with the proximal ones, distal first metatarsal osteotomies have been proved to be simpler and more stable, but with lower correction capability.[15–18] They are recommended generally for only minor and moderate deformities, with less than 50% lateral displacement of the distal fragment in relation to the metatarsal shaft, to insure stability, and to avoid delayed union or malunion.[19–21]

Moreover, it has been more and more recognized that hallux valgus is more than a kind of monoplanar deformity characterized by increased IMA and HVA on a horizontal plane, or a kind of biplanar deformity with abnormal DMAA on sagittal plane as well. In many cases, the deformity is a multiplanar one, with first metatarsal valgus on horizontal plane, enlarged DMAA on sagittal plane, and/or pronation of the first metatarsal on coronal plane.[22–27] In such cases, in order to obtain a 3-dimensionally congruent MTP joint, more complicated and difficult multiplanar or multisite osteotomies other than a monoplanar osteotomy need to be performed. Percutaneous first metatarsal osteotomies are still being performed in China with a linear or a distal oblique closing wedge

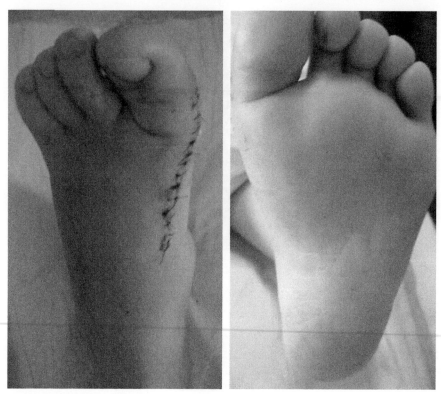

Fig. 25. Immediate postoperative views of the dorsal and plantar surfaces. Note the varus deformity being well corrected.

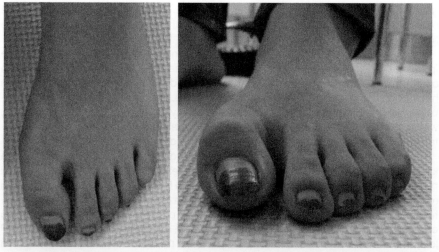

Fig. 26. One-year postoperative views of the dorsal surface. Note the slight dorsal flexion of the MTP joint and the obvious plantar flexion of the IP joint of the great toe.

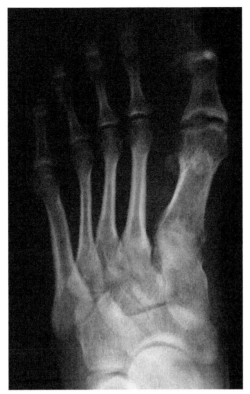

Fig. 27. One-year postoperative AP view of the left foot. Note the arthritis changes in both MTP joint and IP joint.

osteotomy on the head or distal metaphysis site of the first metatarsal. The main differences between percutaneous procedures and traditional open surgeries are the approaches and tools that they use. Percutaneous osteotomies are performed "blindly" and "closely" through tiny approaches with special power rotary burs, whereas traditional open osteotomies are done under direct visualization with saw blades.

The use of percutaneous techniques to perform first metatarsal osteotomy remains a controversial topic. Percutaneous surgeries were proved to have many relative advantages of being less invasive over traditional surgeries,[28–32] but also with inherent drawbacks of less inaccurate and higher demand due to the limitation of narrow working space.[33–35] However, this depends on the type and method of fixation. In most developed countries today where minimally invasive or percutaneous surgeries are performed,[7,31] internal fixation is used to stabilize the osteotomies and prevent many of the complications discussed above.

Reported Outcomes and Some Drawbacks of Percutaneous of the First Metatarsal

Currently, several reports in favor of the unfixed percutaneous first metatarsal osteotomy provide readers with promising and successful results and very few complications. Magnan and colleagues[33] observed clinical and radiographic outcomes in 118 cases of percutaneous distal metatarsal osteotomies from 1996 to 2001 with a mean follow-up of 35.9 months postoperatively. They reported a 91% (107/118) satisfaction rate, an averaging postoperative 88.2 ± 12.9 American Orthopaedic Foot and Ankle

Society (AOFAS) score, and a significant radiographic change (P<.05) (HVA, IMA, DMAA, sesamoid position). In their study, the complications were very few, with only 3 recurrences (2.5%), 8 stiff but not painful first MTP joints (6.8%), and one deep infection (0.8%). The investigators of that study concluded that percutaneous distal osteotomy for correction of hallux valgus was reliable and comparable to traditional surgeries. Mansour and his colleagues[36] reported, in a randomly controlled study with percutaneous surgeries being performed in 31 feet and distal chevron surgeries being performed in 33 feet, that percutaneous distal metatarsal osteotomy had similar clinical and radiological outcomes with distal chevron osteotomy that was performed openly. The complications of the percutaneous osteotomy in their study were only 2/29 (6.9%) pin-track infection. They considered this technique to be a reliable one in treating mild to moderate hallux valgus deformities with good functional and radiological results and high satisfaction. Faour-Martín and colleagues[37] did a prospective study with the retrocapital metatarsal percutaneous osteotomy in 115 feet, with 20° to 40° HVA and up to 20° IMA. Ten-years follow-up results demonstrated that those cases got an improvement of 42.2 points in AOFAS, and HVA was maintained below 20°, with a mean IMA of 8.1°. Complications were 3 skin irritations of K-wire (2.6%), 2 deep infections (1.7%), and 16 limited motility (less than 30° of the MTP joint; 13.9%). Therefore, they concluded that this procedure was effective in mild to moderate deformity in the long term. Enan and colleagues[38] demonstrated in a prospective study in 24 patients that percutaneous distal osteotomy with K-wire fixation got a 31/36 satisfaction rate, with 13.1° HVA correction and 5.4° IMA correction on an average of 21-months follow-up. In this study, no complications were reported. There were no nonunion, malunion, overcorrection, transfer metatarsalgia, or osteonecrosis.

Although the above study results were very promising, most of these studies were uncontrolled case series, with lower-level scientific evidence. In fact, there are very few published high-quality studies giving strong scientific support for these kinds of techniques.[39] There have been also many complications being reported. De Prado and colleagues[40] described 100% shortening of the first metatarsal, 3% displacement of the osteotomy, and 8% delayed union. Weinberger and colleagues[9] performed a retrospective review of 301 percutaneous, unfixed first metatarsal osteotomies for treating hallux valgus that revealed a mean first metatarsal shortening of 5.8 mm ± 2.6 mm, 47 dorsal malunions (15.6%), 11 infections (3.7%), 7 second metatarsal stress fractures (2.3%), 4 delayed unions (1.2%), and 1 hallux varus (0.3%). De Giorgi and colleagues[41] studied 27 consecutive feet operated using Bosch technique at an average follow-up of 19 months (6 months to 5 years). They observed good results in the immediate postoperative time, but all patients had worse radiographic measurements at follow-up. However, they were clinically satisfied, and only one nonunion was recorded.

Kadakia and colleagues[42] originally planned to do a prospective institutional review board–approved study of the percutaneous osteotomy technique. However, the study was halted 3 months later when significant and serious complications with a high rate of recurrence and dorsal malunion were recognized. The 13 mild-to-moderate hallux valgus deformities cases, averaging 130 (range 50–207) days follow-up visit, revealed that 9 cases (69%) developed dorsally angulated malunion with 15.9°; 1 case developed cystic changes consistent with osteonecrosis; 1 case developed a nonunion at 180 days, and 5 cases (38%) were found with recurrence (greater than 15°). Therefore, the investigators came to the conclusion that percutaneous distal metatarsal osteotomy for hallux valgus was associated with an unacceptable rate of complications, specifically, osteonecrosis, nonunion, malunion, and recurrence. The intraoperative correction was routinely lost after removal of the intramedullary Kirschner wire, leading to a high rate of recurrence of hallux valgus deformity as well as dorsal elevation of the capital fragment.

Opponents of this kind of technique point out that the surgery is performed through a very small working window, with most of the treatment being handled "blindly"; therefore, the technique has many unavoidable drawbacks.[39] Most of the published studies show percutaneous surgeries are only indicated for the correction of mild-to-moderate deformity.[32,36–38,43] Furthermore, from the point of view of fixation, in percutaneous surgeries, neither the internally inserted K-wire nor the externally applied bandage dressing could guarantee a safe stabilization of an aggressive osteotomy translation.[9,42] Therefore, percutaneous osteotomy is not indicated for severe deformities. Second, it is not very accurate and could not be adjusted during operation. In percutaneous surgeries, it is impossible to see any anatomy structures through a millimeter-long approach. All treatments are performed without direct visualization. On one hand, "blind" performing is associated with inaccuracy, poor repeatability, and long learning curve. The surgeon is often unable to control the magnitude of translation and rotation. On the other hand, the osteotomy can only be planned, checked, and guided according to radiological examined results. It is gradually realized that the valgus deformity of the big toe is a 3-dimensional one, and the present 2-dimensional radiological evaluation has its own limitations. Recently, it was proved in several studies that frontal plane rotation of the first metatarsal affects the radiological measurements of IMA angle and tibial sesamoid position.[22–27] Therefore, intraoperative evaluation of the actual deformity extent and adjustment of the surgical planning accordingly under direct visualization will definitely increase the accuracy and clinical outcomes of the correction. Third, it is not suitable for complicated cases. In adult patients, not only the deformity but also the degenerative changes of the MTP joint need to be evaluated and treated during operation, such as osteophyte, osteochondral lesion, hypertrophied bunion, and contracture of soft tissue. All these problems could not be well solved percutaneously. Fourth, the osteotomy itself and the fixation are not stable enough. The transverse osteotomy is instable inherently. It is found that even internal fixation with 2 crossing K-wires is insufficient to keep strong stability,[42] not to mention those surgeries with only bandage application and without any internal fixation. In the prospective study, Kadakia and colleagues[42] evaluated the short-term radiographic results and complications of a percutaneous distal metatarsal osteotomy for hallux valgus in 13 patients. They reported that 9 patients (69%) demonstrated a dorsally angulated malalignment at 2 weeks postoperative examination averaging 10.8° (6° to 15°). Those patients had a significant ($P<.0197$) increase in their dorsal malalignment to 15.9° (10° to 22°) at the final 6 weeks follow-up examination after removal of the intramedullary K-wire. Fifth, sufficient soft tissue balancing cannot be achieved in this technique. In traditional open procedures, hallux valgus deformities are always corrected by osseous realignment surgery, combining with soft tissue rebalancing techniques, that is releasing the lateral soft tissue and tightening the medial soft structure. In percutaneous surgeries, it is impossible to perform a medial capsular plication through a minimally invasive approach, which may contribute to the loss of correction and recurrence.

Those disadvantages that are described above may lead to potential complications, including insufficient correction, shortening of first metatarsal, stiffness and/or arthritis of the first MTP joint, transfer metatarsalgia, as well as malunion and nonunion.

Complications of Percutaneous Osteotomy on First Metatarsal that the Authors Met in China and Treatment Option

In the mainland of China, percutaneous osteotomies performed on the first metatarsal are popular, with encouraging outcomes being reported. The real complication rate of this technique in China has been unclear. Although the authors never performed these kinds of surgeries in their practice, in the past 10 years, they have encountered many percutaneous surgeries and treated cases with very poor outcomes and intractable complications.

Shortening/elevation of first metatarsal, transfer metatarsalgia

Because of the limitation of the working approach, percutaneous osteotomy can only be realized with a special rod-shaped rotary burr other than a thin saw blade. The diameter of the burr is about 2 mm, which is much thicker than that of a saw blade (the thinnest blade is 0.4 mm in thickness). However, in addition to the thickness inherent in the burr size, there is also slight bone necrosis on either side of the metatarsal leading to an even greater degree of bone loss. Then, added to this inherent complication of the burr thickness is the angle of the osteotomy, and if the osteotomy is inclined proximally, even more shortening will occur in the metatarsal. Moreover, in cases of attempted correction of more complex deformity with multiplantar osteotomy or rotational displacement, the shortening risk will be even higher. The shortening problem was recognized by De Prado and colleagues,[40] who described a 100% rate of first metatarsal shortening after percutaneous surgery, but did not mention subsequent symptoms.

The shortened first metatarsal is relatively dysfunctional, and more load will be transferred to the lateral metatarsal heads, causing callosity and metatarsalgia. Patients often complain of a painful callosity under the second or more metatarsal heads with difficulty in weight-bearing or walking.[44–46] This problem was well demonstrated in case 1 through case 7. Significant shortening of the first metatarsal with obvious painful callosity under lateral metatarsals caused by transferred loading could be found in those cases. Schemitsch and Horne[47] concluded that a relative ratio of first metatarsal length compared with the second metatarsal length of less than 0.825% might cause symptomatic metatarsalgia.

In planning revision surgery, one must choose either lengthening the first metatarsal or shortening the lateral lesser metatarsals, or both. Each method has its limitations. The short first metatarsal can be lengthened by step-cut osteotomy, open wedge osteotomy, or external fixator distraction. The main postoperative problem of any lengthening is the high compression of the first MTP joint,[48,49] which will cause stiffness, high load, or even arthritis. Just as in the case shown in **Fig. 28**, there is good salvage with nice alignment, but overcompression of the joint and early arthritis also developed. To avoid these problems, sometimes lengthening the EHL tendon and proximal phalanx shortening through Akin osteotomy must be performed as the authors did in case 7. Through reverse Akin osteotomy, they not only decompressed the high pressure on the first MTP joint caused by first metatarsal lengthening but also reinforced the correction of the varus deformity by osseous procedure. In a case with arthrofibrosis or early arthritis of the MTP joint, lengthening the first metatarsal is contraindicated,[48] and an arthrodesis of the MTP joint with or without shortening of the lateral metatarsals is recommended (case 3 and case 4). The authors would like to lengthen the first metatarsal without doing anything to the lesser MTP joints for young patients if the lateral MTP joints are normal.

Shortening osteotomies of the lateral metatarsals using a Weil or the Maceira technique are always used for treating transfer metatarsalgia.[44,50] However, these surgeries also have their inherent complications. The Weil osteotomy can cause a high rate of stiffness (36%) and a floating toe deformity with the toe lying in an extension position and not touching the ground.[50] Sometimes, in the case of a very short first metatarsal, especially with hammer toe deformities and significant symptoms in lesser

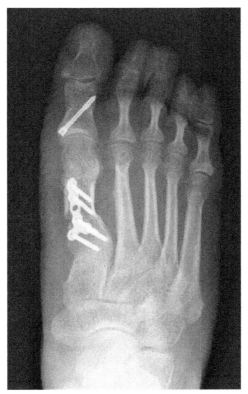

Fig. 28. Lengthening of the first metatarsal bone with nice alignment. Note arthritis of the MTP joint due to overcompression.

toes, lengthening the first metatarsal and shortening the lateral ones need to be combined (case 5)

Elevation of the first metatarsal is another reason of transfer metatarsalgia. It can be caused by dorsal malunion of the osteotomy, or by dysfunction of the stiff or painful first MTP joint. It is often concomitant with shortening of the first metatarsal (case 1 and case 5). The treatment method is to perform a plantar flexion osteotomy.

Stiff first metatarsophalangeal joint
Postoperative stiffness of the first MTP joint is one of the most common complications after hallux valgus surgery.[32,51–54] It can be caused by arthrofibrosis as discussed earlier, too tight a capsulorrhaphy, joint incongruence, or the presence of unrecognized arthritis.[43,51,55] **Fig. 29** is a typical case of overcorrection, causing iatrogenic hallux varus, stiffness, and arthritis. For the right foot, the salvage treatment can be done with medial close wedge osteotomy like Reverdin osteotomy, but that will shorten the first metatarsal again and worsen the IMA as well. Bunionectomy and osteotomy performed with minimally invasive techniques has a high incidence of arthrofibrosis. Although this is should be an extra-articular procedure, which will not cause severe arthrofibrosis or soft tissue contracture, in practice this is not the case, and all are intra-articular procedures that may produce many osseous fragments in the joint and capsular tissues. Although routinely the joint is cleaned with rasps and saline irrigation, there is still high potential of fibrosis caused by residual microscopic fragments, which will lead to pain and stiffness.[39,43,55,56]

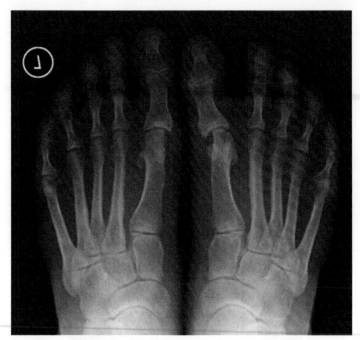

Fig. 29. Overcorrection of Hallux valgus with percutaneous osteotomy. Note the iatrogenic varus and instable first MTP joints.

In treating contracture- or fibrosis-caused joint stiffness, early postoperative mobilization and manipulation can provide some help, but this depends on the stability of the osteotomy, because manipulation of the MTP joint too early will loosen up the osteotomy. It has been the authors' experience that any joint manipulation should be performed within 4 weeks following surgery. Manipulation is followed by injection of corticosteroid and early physical therapy treatment. There is no point to a manipulation in the presence of a malunion of the metatarsal, and an open procedure must be performed that will obtain alignment but may shorten the first metatarsal again.

Painful degenerative first metatarsophalangeal joint

Painful degenerative first MTP joint is often seen in an incongruent joint with aggressive osteotomy. It can also be seen in the case of first metatarsal head necrosis. However, the latter complication is very rare but happens in percutaneous surgeries.[42,48]

Arthrodesis of the first MTP joint is the most standard and reliable treatment. In the case of a very short first metatarsal or a large bone defect after debridement of the dead bone, structural bone block is needed in the fusion.

Fig. 30 is a case of avascular necrosis of the first metatarsal head after operation of percutaneous surgery. The cause of this problem is unclear, possibly due to the instability of the osteotomy and early ambulation. For this case, the only salvage treatment is arthrodesis of the first MTP joint with debridement and bone block transplantation.

Insufficient correction

Reasons for insufficient correction can be divided into 2 groups. One group is due to poor surgical planning and performance. For example, treating cases with enlarged IMA with only lateral tissue release and medial bunionectomy (**Fig. 31**), or just performing the Reverdin-Isham osteotomy.[43,57]

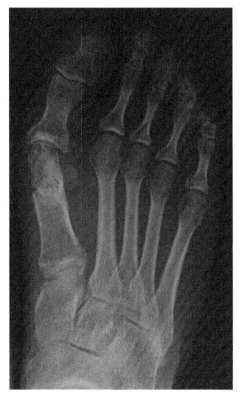

Fig. 30. Avascular necrosis of the first metatarsal head after operation of percutaneous surgery.

Another reason for recurrence of the deformity is due to loss of correction following removal of the percutaneous fixation. Kadakia and colleagues[42] reported a high rate of recurrence (38%) with greater than 15° final HVA at 6 weeks' postoperative follow-up after removal of the K-wire fixation. Revision methods for the insufficient correction are to perform an open osteotomy with adequate soft tissue balance (**Fig. 32**).

Delayed union or nonunion of the osteotomy
This kind of complication is quite common in percutaneous surgeries because of the lack of adequate fixation and primary bone healing. Theoretically, the union rate of this technique should be very high because there is minimal soft tissue stripping. Bösch and colleagues,[6] Giannini and colleagues,[31] and Magnan and colleagues[32] demonstrated very satisfying union rates in their studies, but in a series of cases performed after that of Magnan and Giannini, Kadakia and colleagues[42] came out with totally different study results. Three months after the beginning, their study was stopped because of a high rate of recognized complications. In that study with 13 cases being observed, 1 of 13 cases of nonunion and 9 of 13 cases of dorsal malunion due to the lack of adequate fixation of the osteotomy were reported. The investigators considered this phenomenon needed to be notified because multiple studies demonstrated a 0% nonunion rate after a chevron osteotomy even when combined with a lateral release. The exact cause of the nonunion is unknown. They thought maybe that

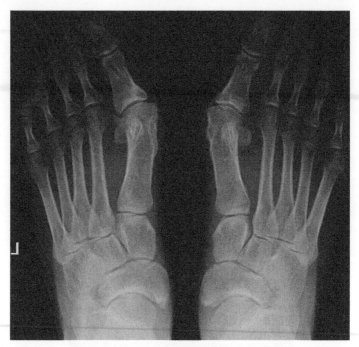

Fig. 31. Insufficient correction with percutaneous bunionectomy bilaterally.

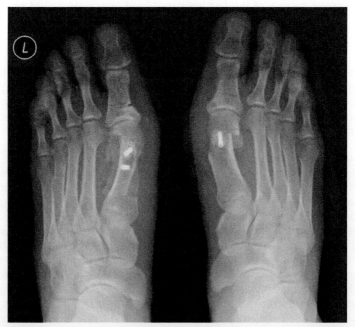

Fig. 32. Immediate AP view after revision surgery. Note the left foot was revised with Scarf and Akin osteotomies, and the right foot was revised with chevron osteotomy.

was the inherent instability of the transverse osteotomy leading to excessive motion at the osteotomy site and an increased risk of nonunion.

At present in the mainland of China, most of the percutaneous osteotomies are still performed without any internal fixation. Therefore, the delayed union or nonunion rate may be even higher. However, there is unfortunately no information reported on the outcome of these treatments.

Hallux varus

Iatrogenic hallux varus is caused by overcorrection or malunion of the osteotomy.[58,59] In planning for revision, one can consider doing the osteotomy again combining with reinforcing the lateral soft tissue structures.[60,61] However, that will have a high risk of causing high compression of the first MTP joint and subsequent arthritis, because in correcting the varus deformity, shortening and/or elevation of the first metatarsal need to be corrected as well. Just as what the authors showed in case 7, after lengthening the first metatarsal with structural bone graft, the varus deformity got even worse, so a reverse Akin osteotomy on the lateral side of the proximal phalanx of the great toe combining with EHB transfer was performed. The only option for treating rigid hallux varus is to perform an arthrodesis of the hallux MTP joint. There are limited mobility, arthrofibrosis or arthritis, and deformity of the first MTP joint, and MTP arthrodesis is a good and more reliable procedure.[62]

Moreover, improper performance due to the low repeatability of the percutaneous osteotomy technique may also be considered as one cause of those above-mentioned complications.[33–35]

SUMMARY

Percutaneous osteotomies of the first metatarsal do have several advantages, like minimal surgical trauma, short operating time, and quicker recovery. However, they are also in high demand on the performance and indication selection. They need to be handled by senior surgeons who are familiar with both open and percutaneous methods of treatment, following comprehensive evaluation of the cases, very strict indication selection, and extensive training in the procedure. Otherwise, incorrect usage will bring intractable complications.

Revision of these complications can be very difficult and associated with uncertain long-term results. Complications of percutaneous surgery of the first metatarsal can generally be predictably corrected with arthrodesis of the first MTP joint. Although alternative techniques, such as open osteotomies and/or shortening osteotomies of the lesser metatarsals, are options, in order to provide a stable medial column, arthrodesis should be the best treatment of choice in cases where substantial bone has been lost.

SUPPLEMENTARY DATA

Supplementary data related to this article can be found at http://dx.doi.org/10.1016/j.fcl.2016.04.011.

REFERENCES

1. Hymes L. Introduction: brief history of the use of minimum incision surgery (MIS). In: Fielding MD, editor. Forefoot minimum incision in podiatric medicine: a handbook on primary corrective procedures on the human foot using minimum incisions with minimum trauma. New York: Futura Pub Co; 1977. p. 1–2.

2. Van Enoo RE, Cane EM. Minimal incision surgery: a plastic technique or a cover-up? Clin Podiatr Med Surg 1986;5:485–98.

3. David C, Sammarco G, James G. Minimum incision surgery. Foot Ankle Int 1992; 13:157–60.

4. Gorechi GA, Weissman S, Kidawa AS. Lixiscope: a podiatric evaluation. J Am Podiatry Assoc 1982;72:304–6.

5. Hohmann G. Symptomatische oder physiologische Behandlung des Hallux valgus. Munch Med Wochenschr 1921;68:1042–5 [in German].

6. Bösch P, Wanke S, Legenstein R. Hallux valgus correction by the method of Bösch: a new technique with a seven-to-ten-year follow-up. Foot Ankle Clin 2000;5:485–98.

7. Bösch P, Markowski H, Rannicher V. Technik und erste Ergebnisse der subkuta-nen distalen Metatarsale-I-Osteotomie. Orthopaedische Praxis 1990;26:51–6 [in German].

8. Lamprecht E, Kramer J. Die Metatarsale-I-Osteotomie nach Kramer zur Behand-lung des Hallux valgus. Orthopaedische Praxis 1982;28:635–45 [in German].

9. Weinberger BH, Fulp JM, Falstrom P, et al. Retrospective evaluation of percuta-neous bunionectomies and distal osteotomies without internal fixation. Clin Po-diatr Med Surg 1991;8:111–36.

10. Myerson MS, Komenda GA. Results of hallux varus correction using an extensor hallucis brevis tenodesis. Foot Ankle Int 1996;17:21–7.

11. Lucijanic I, Bicanic G, Sonicki Z, et al. Treatment of hallux valgus with three-dimensional modification of Mitchell's osteotomy: technique and results. J Am Po-diatr Med Assoc 2009;99:162–72.

12. Mitchell CL, Fleming JL, Allen R, et al. Osteotomy-bunionectomy for hallux valgus. J Bone Joint Surg Am 1958;40:41–58.

13. Wilson JN. Oblique displacement osteotomy for hallux valgus. J Bone Joint Surg Br 1963;45:552–6.

14. Grace DL. Metatarsal osteotomy: which operation? J Foot Surg 1987;26:46–50.

15. Wagner E, Ortiz C. Osteotomy considerations in hallux valgus treatment: improving the correction power. Foot Ankle Clin 2012;17:481–98.

16. Trnka HJ. Osteotomies for hallux valgus correction. Foot Ankle Clin 2005;10: 15–33.

17. Nyska M. Principles of first metatarsal osteotomies. Foot Ankle Clin 2001;6: 399–408.

18. Easley ME, Trnka HJ. Current concepts review: hallux valgus part II: operative treatment. Foot Ankle Int 2007;28:748–58.

19. Hattrup SJ, Johnson KA. Chevron osteotomy: analysis of factors of patients' dissatisfaction. Foot Ankle Int 1985;5:327–32.

20. Mann RA, Coughlin MJ. Adult hallux valgus. In: Coughlin MJ, Mann RA, editors. Surgery of the foot and ankle. 7th edition. St Louis (MO): Mosby; 1999. p. 150–269.

21. Meier PJ, Kenzora JE. The risks and benefits of distal first metatarsal osteoto-mies. Foot Ankle Int 1985;6:7–17.

22. Chi TD, Davitt J, Younger A, et al. Intra- and inter-observer reliability of the distal metatarsal articular angle in adult hallux valgus. Foot Ankle Int 2002;23:722–6.

23. Coughlin MJ, Freund E. Roger A. Mann award. The reliability of angular measure-ments in hallux valgus deformities. Foot Ankle Int 2001;22:369–79.

24. Lee KM, Ahn S, Chung CY, et al. Reliability and relationship of radiographic mea-surements in hallux valgus. Clin Orthop Relat Res 2012;470:2613–21.

25. Mortier JP, Bernard JL, Maestro M. Axial rotation of the first metatarsal head in a normal population and hallux valgus patients. Orthop Traumatol Surg Res 2012; 98:677–83.
26. Dayton P, Feilmeier M, Hirschi J, et al. Observed changes in radiographic measurements of the first ray after frontal plane rotation of the first metatarsal in a cadaveric foot model. J Foot Ankle Surg 2014;53:274–8.
27. Park CH, Cho JH, Moon JJ, et al. Can double osteotomy be a solution for adult hallux valgus deformity with an increased distal metatarsal articular angle? J Foot Ankle Surg 2016;55(1):188–92.
28. LÓpez JJG, RodrÍguez SR, Méndez LC. Functional, esthetic and radiographic results of treatment of hallux valgus with minimally invasive surgery. Acta Orthop Mex 2005;19:S42–6.
29. Migues A, Campaner G, Slullitel G, et al. Minimally invasive surgery in hallux valgus and digital deformities. Orthopedics 2007;30:523–6.
30. Leemrijse T, Valtin B, Besse JL. Hallux valgus surgery in 2005. Conventional, mini-invasive or percutaneous surgery? Uni- or bilateral? Hospitalization or one-day surgery? Rev Chir Orthop Reparatrice Appar Mot 2008;94(2):111–27.
31. Giannini S, Faldini C, Vannini F, et al. The minimally invasive osteotomy "S.E.R.I." (simple, effective, rapid, inexpensive) for correction of bunionette deformity. Foot Ankle Int 2008;29:282–6.
32. Portaluri M. Hallux valgus correction by the method of Bösch: a clinical evaluation. Foot Ankle Clin 2000;5:499–511.
33. Magnan B, Pezzè L, Rossi N, et al. Percutaneous distal metatarsal osteotomy for correction of hallux valgus. J Bone Joint Surg Am 2005;87:1191–9.
34. Roukis TS. Percutaneous and minimum incision metatarsal osteotomies: a systematic review. J Foot Ankle Surg 2009;48:380–7.
35. Roukis TS. Central metatarsal head-neck osteotomies: indications and operative techniques. Clin Podiatr Med Surg 2005;22:197–222.
36. Roukis TS, Schade VL. Minimum-incision metatarsal osteotomies. Clin Podiatr Med Surg 2008;25:587–607.
37. Radwan YA, Mansour AM. Percutaneous distal metatarsal osteotomy versus distal chevron osteotomy for correction of mild-to-moderate hallux valgus deformity. Arch Orthop Trauma Surg 2012;132:1539–46.
38. Faour-Martín O, Martín-Ferrero MA, Valverde García JA, et al. Long-term results of the retrocapital metatarsal percutaneous osteotomy for hallux valgus. Int Orthop 2013;37:1799–803.
39. Enan A, Abo-Hegy M, Seif H. Early results of distal metatarsal osteotomy through minimally invasive approach for mild-to-moderate hallux valgus. Acta Orthop Belg 2010;76:526–35.
40. Maffulli N, Longo UG, Marinozzi A, et al. Hallux valgus: effectiveness and safety of minimally invasive surgery. A systematic review. Br Med Bull 2011;97:149–67.
41. De Prado M, Ripoll PL, Vaquero J, et al. Tratamiento quirurgico per cutaneo del hallux mediante osteotomias multiples. Rev Orthop Traumatol 2003;47:406–16 [in Spanish].
42. De Giorgi S, Mascolo V, Losito A. The correction of hallux valgus by Bösch technique (PDO—Percutaneous Distal Osteotomy). GIOT 2003;29:161–4.
43. Kadakia AR, Smerek JP, Myerson MS. Radiographic results after percutaneous distal metatarsal osteotomy for correction of hallux valgus deformity. Foot Ankle Int 2007;28:355–60.
44. Bauer T, de Lavigne C, Biau D, et al. Percutaneous hallux valgus surgery: a prospective multicenter study of 189 cases. Orthop Clin North Am 2009;40:505–14.

45. Maceira E, Monteagudo M. Transfer metatarsalgia post hallux valgus surgery. Foot Ankle Clin 2014;19:285–307.
46. Lehman DE. Salvage of complications of hallux valgus surgery. Foot Ankle Clin 2003;8:15–35.
47. Espinosa N, Brodsky JW, Maceira E. Metatarsalgia. J Am Acad Orthop Surg 2010;18:474–85.
48. Schemitsch E, Horne G. Wilson's osteotomy for the treatment of hallux valgus. Clin Orthop Relat Res 1989;240:221–5.
49. Goldberg A, Singh D. Treatment of shortening following hallux valgus surgery. Foot Ankle Clin 2014;19:309–16.
50. Siekmann W, Watson TS, Roggelin M. Correction of moderate to severe hallux valgus with isometric first metatarsal double osteotomy. Foot Ankle Int 2014;35: 1122–30.
51. Klinge SA, McClure P, Fellars T, et al. Modification of the Weil/Maceira metatarsal osteotomy for coronal plane malalignment during crossover toe correction: case series. Foot Ankle Int 2014;35:584–91.
52. Schneider W, Aigner N, Pinggera O, et al. Chevron osteotomy in hallux valgus: ten-year results of 112 cases. J Bone Joint Surg Br 2004;86:1016–20.
53. Freslon M, Gayet LE, Bouche G, et al. Scarf osteotomy for the treatment of hallux valgus: a review of 123 cases with 4.8 years follow-up. Rev Chir Orthop Reparatrice Appar Mot 2005;91:257–66 [in French].
54. Jones CP, Coughlin MJ, Grebing BR, et al. First metatarsophalangeal joint motion after hallux valgus correction: a cadaver study. Foot Ankle Int 2005;26:614–9.
55. Skoták M, Behounek J. Scarf osteotomy for the treatment of forefoot deformity. Acta Chir Orthop Traumatol Cech 2006;73:18–22 [in Czech].
56. Isham SA. The Reverdin–Isham procedure for the correction of hallux abducto valgus. A distal metatarsal osteotomy procedure. Clin Podiatr Med Surg 1991; 8:81–94.
57. Markowski HP, Bosch P, Rannicher V. Surgical technique and preliminary results of percutaneous neck osteotomy of the first metatarsal for hallux valgus. Foot 1992;2:93–8.
58. Bauer T. Percutaneous forefoot surgery. Orthop Traumatol Surg Res 2014;100: S191–204.
59. Crawford MD, Patel J, Giza E. Iatrogenic hallux varus treatment algorithm. Foot Ankle Clin 2014;19:371–84.
60. Davies MB, Blundell CM. The treatment of iatrogenic hallux varus. Foot Ankle Clin 2014;19:275–84.
61. Plovanich EJ, Donnenwerth MP, Abicht BP, et al. Failure after soft-tissue release with tendon transfer for flexible iatrogenic hallux varus: a systematic review. J Foot Ankle Surg 2012;51:195–7.
62. Geaney LE, Myerson MS. Radiographic results after hallux metatarsophalangeal joint arthrodesis for hallux varus. Foot Ankle Int 2015;36:391–4.

Percutaneous Surgery for Metatarsalgia and the Lesser Toes

David J. Redfern, FRCS (Tr&Orth)[a],*, Joel Vernois, MD[b]

KEYWORDS

- Percutaneous • Distal metatarsal metaphyseal osteotomies (DMMO) • Metatarsalgia
- Hammertoe • Minimally invasive surgery

KEY POINTS

- The traditional open surgical options for the treatment of metatarsalgia and lesser toe deformities are limited and often result in unintentional stiffness.
- The use of percutaneous techniques for the treatment of metatarsalgia and lesser toe deformities allows a more versatile and tailor-made approach to the individual deformities.
- As with all percutaneous techniques, it is vital the surgeon engage in cadaveric training from surgeons experienced in these techniques before introducing them into his/her clinical practice.

METATARSALGIA

Metatarsalgia means pain in the region of the metatarsal heads and is obviously not a diagnosis but a symptom for which there can be many causes and often several contributing factors. This concept might seem simple, but the complaint can be anything but simple to adequately explain and successfully treat.

The treating clinician must possess an in-depth understanding of the mechanics of the foot and ankle and the disease processes affecting these extremities. A detailed clinical assessment is required to ascertain the relevant cause or causes of the complaint. Only by understanding the relevant cause or causes of metatarsalgia in a patient can the clinician hope to offer a successful long-term treatment solution.

These principles remain the same whether contemplating traditional open or percutaneous surgical treatment. This article focuses on the role of percutaneous surgical options in the treatment of metatarsalgia and hence focuses on surgical alteration of the metatarsal cascade via metatarsal osteotomy and correction of frequently associated lesser toe deformities.

The authors have nothing to disclose.

[a] The London Foot & Ankle Centre, Hospital St John & St Elizabeth, 60 Grove End Road, St John's Wood, London NW8 9NH, UK; [b] Brighton & Sussex University Hospitals Trust, Princess Royal Hospital, Lewes Road, Haywards Heath, West Sussex, RH16 4EY, UK
* Corresponding author.
E-mail address: david.redfern@springgroup.org

Foot Ankle Clin N Am 21 (2016) 527–550
http://dx.doi.org/10.1016/j.fcl.2016.04.003
1083-7515/16/$ – see front matter © 2016 Elsevier Inc. All rights reserved.

foot.theclinics.com

It should be stressed that the surgical treatment of metatarsalgia frequently does *not* require lesser metatarsal osteotomies, and the authors consider such osteotomies (whether performed open or minimally invasively) to be a last port of call rather than a first. For example, the vast majority of patients presenting with metatarsalgia of primarily mechanical rather than biological etiology have an associated hallux valgus deformity. In most of these cases, correction of the hallux valgus with adequate triplanar displacement of corrective first metatarsal osteotomy will be sufficient to abolish the metatarsalgia symptoms (without recourse to lesser metatarsal osteotomies), refunctioning the windlass mechanism and improving load distribution in the forefoot.

Distal Lesser Metatarsal Osteotomies

The Weil osteotomy has for many years remained the most popular lesser metatarsal osteotomy for treating abnormalities of the metatarsal cascade/imbalance of load distribution across the forefoot. However, although broadly adopted by foot and ankle surgeons, Weil osteotomy has a high incidence of postoperative stiffness and floating toe,[1,2] and it is very difficult to create and fix these osteotomies with correct metatarsal length *and* sagittal profile for the unique mechanics of a particular patient. The work of Maestro and colleagues[3] has been widely adopted as a method for calculating appropriate metatarsal length and hence position of fixation for Weil osteotomies but fails to take into account the sagittal plane of the metatarsal (metatarsal inclination; **Fig. 1**) and other relevant mechanical factors, such as the overall architecture of the foot, ankle motion, gastrocsoleus tension, and the functional needs of the individual patient (footwear and so on). Khurna and colleagues,[4] who correlated poor outcome following Weil osteotomy with sagittal plane imbalance on a metatarsal skyline view,

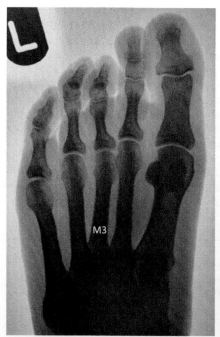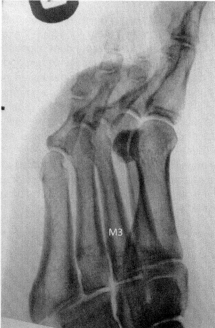

Fig. 1. In the AP view (*left*), the third metatarsal (M3) appears short, but in the oblique view (*right*), it is clear that it is apparent shortening due to increased plantar obliquity of the ray.

demonstrated the importance of considering the metatarsal sagittal inclination in avoiding poor results. Hence, the idea of avoiding fixation of lesser metatarsal osteotomies rigidly with internal fixation and allowing a "dynamic" correction with controlled movement/settlement according to the mechanical environment is appealing.

Distal Metatarsal Metaphyseal Osteotomies

The term distal metatarsal metaphyseal osteotomies (DMMO) is descriptive of the site of the osteotomy, which in turn, is very important in dictating the behavior of this percutaneous procedure. The DMMO has gained popularity in Europe as an alternative surgical technique to the traditional Weil osteotomy because of the problems observed with stiffness and floating toe with the Weil and because of the perceived potential advantages of a dynamic correction offered by the DMMO.

The DMMO is performed via a tiny portal at the distal diaphyseal-metaphyseal junction of the lesser metatarsal using a Shannon burr (2 × 12 mm) at an angle of 45° to the plane of the metatarsal (**Fig. 2**).

Surgical Technique

Equipment
The equipment used is a Beaver Blade.

Burr A 2 mm × 12 mm Shannon burr is used (Wright Medical, Memphis, USA).

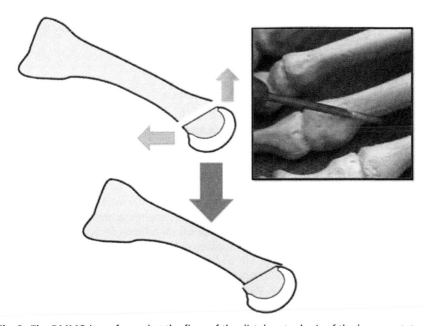

Fig. 2. The DMMO is performed at the flare of the distal metaphysis of the lesser metatarsal at a plane of 45° to the metatarsal axis in the sagittal plane. In making the osteotomy at this level, the amount of dorsal displacement (dictated by weight-bearing forces) is limited by the proximal fragment. The proximal fragment also limits the amount of shortening (dictated by the soft tissue tension). This avoids overcorrection. With experience, the plane can be adjusted to discourage/encourage medial/lateral displacement (also dictated by the soft tissues) and to favor primarily elevation or shortening. The inset shows the correct position of the burr to initiate the cut.

Tourniquet A tourniquet is not required, and use of the tourniquet will prevent bleeding at the portals, which is helpful in cooling the burr (and hence may increase the risk of thermal injury).

Image intensifier An image intensifier is sensible to begin with, but as the surgeon becomes more experienced, it will not be required.

Anesthesia
Either general or regional anesthetic is administered as well as intravenous antibiotics as per local guidelines.

Positioning
The patient is positioned supine with the feet overhanging the end of the table (unless combining with open surgery in which case it is preferable to have the foot stabilized with the heel on the table). The mini C-arm is positioned to the right of the patient whether operating on the left or right foot (position the C-arm on the left side for left-handed surgeon).

DMMO[5]
1. The nondominant hand (NDH) is important as "sat-nav" for positioning the osteotomy. The thumb of the NDH is placed on the dorsal surface of the metatarsophalangeal joint (MTPJ) so that it covers the dorsal articular surface. The index finger of the NDH is placed on the plantar surface of the MTPJ, and hence, the surgeon has the MTPJ between the thumb and index finger. A transverse stab incision is then made with the dominant hand using a Beaver Blade. The incision is placed to the right side of, and adjacent to, the MTPJ (left side if left-handed). The incision is only skin deep, and no deepening/periosteal elevation is required and might risk damaging local the blood supply to the metatarsal head.
2. Then a 12-mm Shannon burr is inserted through the portal and directed extracapsularly toward the right-hand side of the metatarsal neck (left if left-handed). The burr is then firmly rasped on metatarsal neck so as to locate the distal stop-point on the neck, where the burr abuts the capsule of the MTPJ on the distal flare of the metatarsal neck on its right side. This position is where the osteotomy commences at an angle of 45° to the axis of the metatarsal sagittal axis (see **Fig. 2**). The correct starting positioning of the burr can be confirmed on an image intensifier, although this will be unnecessary with experience.
3. The burr is then engaged in the right-hand side of the metatarsal neck at a low speed while maintaining the sagittal 45° angle to the metatarsal axis. As the burr cuts through the cortex on this right side of the metatarsal neck, the surgeon can continue the osteotomy by steadily supinating their wrist in a smooth action until the burr lies flat on the foot at 90° to the metatarsal axis in the anteroposterior (AP) plane (**Fig. 3**A). If the burr does not end up at 90° to the metatarsal axis at completion of the osteotomy, then the surgeon will create an oblique osteotomy (**Fig. 3**B, C).
4. Because of the larger dimensions of the second metatarsal, the surgeon also needs to use a sawing action in addition to the supination motion in order to complete the osteotomy here (otherwise the cutting flutes of the 12-mm Shannon burr are not long enough to cut dorsal and plantar cortices in one sweep). The osteotomy should always finish on the dorsal metatarsal surface exiting just proximal to the thumb of the NDH and in so doing ensuring the osteotomy remains extra-articular.
5. A right-handed surgeon will find it easiest to begin with the fourth metatarsal DMMO in the left foot and then progress to the third, and then the second. In

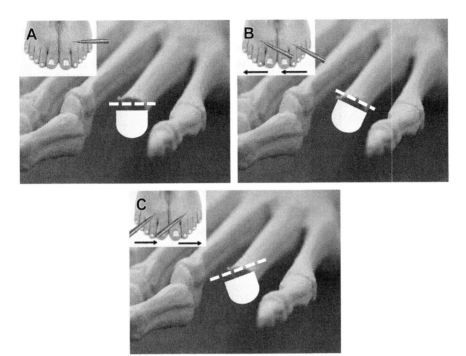

Fig. 3. Effects of altering finishing position of burr hand-piece on plane of osteotomy. (*A*) Correct end-point with burr driver hand-piece perpendicular to the axis of the metatarsal (*inset*). This will result in a perpendicular osteotomy as shown. (*B*) If a right-handed surgeon finishes the osteotomy with the burr hand-piece directed as shown in the inset, then the result will be an oblique metatarsal osteotomy, which will encourage lateralization of the metatarsal head in the right foot but will discourage lateralization in the left foot. (*C*) If a right-handed surgeon finishes the osteotomy with the burr hand-piece directed as shown in the inset, then the result will be an oblique metatarsal osteotomy, which will encourage lateralization of the metatarsal head in the left foot but will discourage lateralization in the right foot.

this way, the fourth metatarsal head will "fall" out of the way before doing the third and so on, allowing more room for the surgeon to create the osteotomy in the next metatarsal. In the right foot, the advice is reversed for a right-handed surgeon (easiest to begin with the second metatarsal, then third, and then fourth).

6. The osteotomy is *only* complete when the metatarsal head is mobile in the sagittal plane *and* also telescopes in a proximal-distal plane. If both these planes of motion are not present, then there will some intact bone-/periosteum-limiting motion and this must be cut and freed.
7. The position of the osteotomy and the plane in which it is made can be significantly altered if the surgeon does not adhere to the technique detailed above. Relatively small changes in the position of the osteotomy and its plane can have large effects on its behavior (see **Fig. 3**; **Fig. 4**).

Postoperative Care

The patient should be told to elevate the operated leg for 45 minutes out of every hour for the first 2 weeks after surgery. The patient should be provided with a stiff-soled

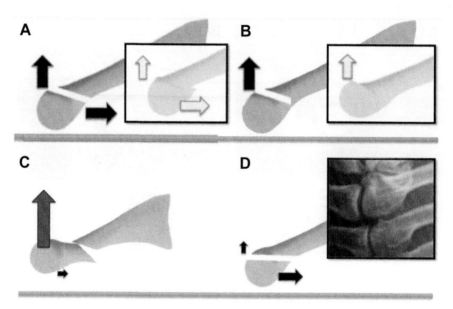

Fig. 4. How positioning of the osteotomy affects its behavior. (*A*) Standard DMMO with complete osteotomy at the flare of the distal metaphysis of the lesser metatarsal. (*B*) Distal (metatarsal) incomplete metaphyseal osteotomy. This is performed in exactly the same position as the standard DMMO but the plantar cortex is not cut. The osteotomy can then be closed (in dorsal direction) to achieve pure elevation of the metatarsal head. This is also an extracapsular osteotomy. (*C*) It is an error to make the osteotomy more proximally because this will completely change the behavior of the osteotomy. The point of rotation of the osteotomy will move proximally and the osteotomy will displace primarily in dorsal rotation, likely resulting in overelevation of the metatarsal head. (*D*) It is an error to make the osteotomy too distally (intracapsular) because this will result in a residual shelf overhang of bone (as the metatarsal head displaces proximally), which can cause stiffness and pain.

postoperative shoe and encouraged to full weight-bear in this immediately as comfort allows. Crutches are provided to provide stability, but as already stated, the patient can safely be allowed to full weight-bear.

Patients should be told that the preoperative metatarsalgia is usually abolished immediately, but that in its place there is often pain on the dorsal aspect of the forefoot initially. In addition, the patient may notice clicking in the forefoot due to movement at the osteotomy sites. They should be reassured in regards the clicking symptoms because they reflect weight-bearing movement of the metatarsal heads, which is desired in this dynamic correction. Veno-thromboembolism prophylaxis should be implemented according to local guidelines.

The patient is reviewed at 2 weeks after surgery, and bandages and dressings are removed at this stage to inspect the portals. Once healed, the portals can be left uncovered, and the patient can be instructed to continue use of the stiff-soled postoperative shoe for a further 4 weeks, at which point they can migrate into their own footwear. Patients should be warned that the postoperative swelling will persist for 4 to 6 months (or occasionally longer with delayed union).

Further outpatient review usually takes place at 6 to 8 weeks after surgery and then at 4 to 6 months after surgery. Once wearing their own footwear, the patient can be allowed to gradually increase their activity level as dictated by their symptoms. However, generally, no return to sport should be allowed before 3 months after surgery. No further radiological review is usually undertaken unless there is persisting swelling and/or discomfort at 6 months after surgery.

Indications/Contraindications

The indications are largely the same as for the Weil osteotomy. Surgeons vary in their threshold to use Weil osteotomies, and as previously stated, lesser metatarsal osteotomies (whether performed with open or percutaneous technique) should be a port of last call rather than first.

Contraindications are also the same as those for the Weil osteotomy, including active infection and insufficient vascular perfusion. However, because of the tiny percutaneous portal incisions, DMMOs can often be considered in situations where there is poor local soft tissue or previous incisions/scarring that might otherwise be of concern with larger open incisions (eg, Weil). Redfern advises against DMMO in the presence of significant arthritis and stiffness in the associated MTPJ because of the observed increased risk of nonunion in this situation (motion then predominantly occurs at the osteotomy site rather than the MTPJ).

When performing DMMOs, it should generally be considered obligatory to perform the osteotomies to the second, third, and fourth metatarsals in order to avoid a transfer lesion developing under the third or fourth metatarsal heads. A DMMO of the fifth should also be added in the presence of a relatively small length difference between fourth and fifth metatarsals to avoid symptoms in the fifth toe where it will not sit comfortably against the fourth toe. Isolated DMMOs of a single metatarsal should generally be avoided but can be undertaken in specific circumstances when very experienced with this technique.

The surgical technique, correct postoperative care, and potential complications have been well described.[5]

Complications

The list of potential complications is the same as for an open osteotomy, including infection (<0.5%), soft tissue complications, delayed/nonunion, and malunion. Symptomatic nonunion is rare (approximately 1:500–1:1000).[5] However, delayed union is in the region of 5% and usually affects the second (or third less commonly) metatarsal osteotomies. In the case of DMMOs, the authors define delayed union as incomplete radiological evidence of union at 6 months after surgery. It is therefore important to warn the patient of this potential complication. Usually the delayed union is hypertrophic, indicating attempted healing in a suboptimal mechanical environment, and if symptomatic, then placing the foot in a short removable boot for 4 to 6 weeks with advice to minimize weight-bearing activity is likely to achieve union. In the vast majority of cases, there will be progression to radiological union by 12 months.

With Weil osteotomies, because of the rigid internal fixation, there is rarely malunion. However, with no internal fixation, DMMOs can displace during the healing period, seemingly due to the force exerted by the extensor hallucis brevis, which can result in lateralization of M2 and M3 and almost always some medialization of the M5 head (advantageous in treating bunionette deformity) (**Fig. 5**). The displacement is not usually significant and rarely compromises the clinical result, but care should be taken when combining DMMOs with hallux valgus correction because the tendency for M2 and M3 lateralization during the postoperative period is increased.

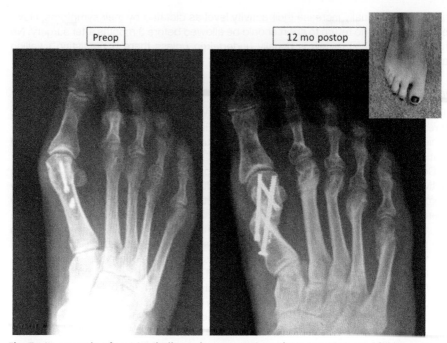

Fig. 5. An example of revision hallux valgus correction. The presenting complaint was predominantly metatarsalgia. A 'minimally invasive chevron akin hallux valgus correction was undertaken in conjunction with DMMOs and percutaneous lesser toe corrections (P1 osteotomies of toes 2 and 3). The tendency for lateralization of the M2 and M3 heads was well controlled by altering the obliquity of the DMMOs (see **Fig. 3**) and by strapping of the lesser toes postoperatively. Note the medialization of the M5 head after DMMO. This is an effective way to treat Redfern type II bunionettes (see **Box 1**).

Results

There is still relatively little comparative literature to draw on when studying the results of this technique, but those studies that are available suggest at least equivalent efficacy when compared with the results of Weil osteotomies in the treatment of metatarsalgia.[6,7] In the opinion of these authors, the lack of postoperative stiffness is the main attraction with DMMOs, but the tradeoff is almost certainly prolonged swelling in some patients and higher incidence of delayed union, although symptoms from this are usually low level. Symptomatic nonunion is rare (<1% in the experience of these authors).

Taylor Bunion/Bunionette

It seems appropriate to mention Taylor bunions at this point, because the treatment of such deformities using these techniques is very simple. A clinical classification of bunionette deformity is preferred over the traditional radiological classification (**Box 1**).[5] The Redfern clinical classification divides these deformities into 2 groups:

Type I: The fifth toe is straight.
Type II: The fifth toe is in varus.
An additional subgroup also (type Ia/IIa) describes associated supination of the fifth toe.

Box 1
Redfern clinical classification of bunionette deformities

Type I: fifth toe straight

- Fifth toe straight is equivalent to radiological type 1 bunionette deformity.

- A simple percutaneous shaving of the prominent fifth metatarsal head can be undertaken and no fifth metatarsal osteotomy is required.

- The patient can full weight-bear immediately and can usually return to normal footwear within the first few days after surgery. Subsequent increase in patient activity can safely be dictated by their comfort.

Type II: fifth toe varus alignment

- Fifth toe varus alignment is equivalent to a radiological type II/III deformity.

- Fifth toe varus alignment requires a fifth metatarsal osteotomy regardless of any oversize of the fifth metatarsal head, and a DMMO of the fifth metatarsal is almost always sufficient to treat these.

- The DMMO will always result in the fifth metatarsal head moving medially due to the axis of the extensor digitorum brevis acting on the fifth toe.

- With severe widening of the 4/5 intermetatarsal angle or severe "banana" deformity of the fifth metatarsal (severe type II and III by radiological classification), the surgeon can use a more proximal closing wedge osteotomy if preferred, but Redfern would still favor a DMMO in such circumstances with trimming of any proximal fragment lateral wall prominence as required.

- Postoperatively the foot can be simply taped (for 4 weeks) to maintain correction.

- Patients can full weight-bear immediately and can usually return to normal footwear after the first postoperative week. Subsequent increase in patient activity can safely be dictated by their comfort.

Type Ia/IIa: additional rotational (supination) deformity of the fifth toe

- Treatment for these deformities begins with a derotation osteotomy of the fifth toe by performing a complete proximal phalanx osteotomy (at the proximal diaphyseal/metaphyseal junction) (see hammer toe section). Treatment then proceeds as described above for the type I/II deformity.

- Postoperatively the fifth toe is taped in the desired rotation for 4 weeks.

Complications

Complications are unusual. Delayed union is rare with DMMO of the fifth metatarsal, and these authors have not encountered nonunion at this site with this technique. As described above, is important to shave down the prominent lateral wall of the fifth metatarsal diaphysis with larger displacements.

If using a more proximal medial closing wedge osteotomy for larger deformities (not necessary in the opinion of these authors), then the surgeon should be aware of the risk of metatarsal elevation in the postoperative period due to the increased moment arm acting on the distal metatarsal.

LESSER TOE DEFORMITIES

Percutaneous surgical techniques are particularly appealing for the correction of lesser toe deformities and may be advantageous in cases considered at higher risk of cutaneous or vascular complications.

The main advantage is that these techniques afford the surgeon an almost limitless "à la carte" menu of surgical options that can be tailored to a particular deformity without the concerns of scar contracture and similar that can be of concern with the limited open armamentarium. Percutaneous correction of these deformities allows targeted soft tissue and bone procedures (of any of the phalanges/joints) for different types of deformity of varying flexibility and reducibility. Operative time-savings should not be the driving concern in embarking on these techniques because although many flexible deformities can be corrected quickly, more complex and fixed deformities with or without subluxation/dislocation can take as long or longer than open surgical techniques.

Surgical Technique

Equipment
Equipment includes minimally invasive instruments, including rasp and straight elevator.

Burr A 2 mm × 8 mm Shannon burr is used (Wright Medical, Memphis, USA).

Tourniquet A tourniquet is not required and may encourage thermal injury to the soft tissues because the cooling effect of hemorrhage at the portals is lost. If undertaking these techniques with a tourniquet, then saline irrigation should be used.

Anesthesia
Either general or regional anesthesia is administered as well as intravenous antibiotics as per local guidelines.

Positioning
The positioning is the same as for DMMO.

Techniques

The surgical techniques for the various types of lesser toe procedures are summarized in **Table 1** and **Fig. 6**. As with open surgical techniques, the way in which the techniques/elements of surgery are used or combined in different clinical situations will vary from surgeon to surgeon, but the Redfern algorithm for the management of hammer toe deformities is detailed in **Fig. 10**.

A list of percutaneous surgical techniques available (**Fig. 7**) includes:
1. Soft tissue procedures
   a. Flexor tenotomies: flexor digitorum brevis, FDB; flexor digitorum longus, FDL
   b. Extensor tenotomies: extensor digitorum longus, EDL; extensor digitorum brevis, EDB
   c. Joint release: metatarsophalangeal; plantar proximal interphalangeal, PIP
2. Bone procedures
   a. Extra-articular: phalangeal osteotomy (proximal phalanx [P1], middle [P2])
   b. Intra-articular: condylectomy, condyloplasty, fusion (PIP, distal interphalangeal [DIP])

Postoperative Management

Any surgeon wishing to take up these techniques must be familiar with techniques to control the toe position in the postoperative period while healing occurs. Generally, wet gauze dressings are used intraoperatively (although the option of K-wires in some cases may be appropriate such as percutaneous plantar proximal interphalangeal joint [PIPJ] fusion). At the first postoperative review (usually 1–2 weeks after

Table 1
Summary of percutaneous techniques for correction of lesser toe deformity

Type	Description	Approach	Summary of Technique	Stabilization	Comments
Soft tissue surgery	FDB tenotomy	Midaxial approach just proximal to PIPJ	The Beaver Blade is introduced to the right side of the toe just proximal to the PIPJ (onto the plantar surface of the distal P1) and translated distally into the PIPJ (releasing the PP). The blade is then advanced onto the undersurface of the P2 and rotated to release both heads of the FDB (blade remaining on the plantar surface of the P2).	Depends on bony surgery; not usually performed in isolation	Neurovascular bundle remains safe as long as the toe is not forcibly straightened while performing the release Useful technique for converting stiff deformities of PIPJ to flexible deformities[5]
	FDL tenotomy	Plantar at level of DIPJ	Longitudinal stab incision into DIPJ and rotate the Beaver Blade left and right while keeping an extension force on the DIPJ; completion of the tenotomy confirmed when there is no resistance to dorsiflexion	Steri-Strip over terminal phalanx of toe to control position if required	Can also be performed in similar fashion to FDB release via a midaxial approach
	EDB tenotomy	Dorsal, proximal to MTPJ	Can be selectively released using a stab incision approximately 2 cm proximal to the MTPJ	Depends on other concurrent procedures to the toe	Preferable to maintain integrity of one of the extensors to avoid defunctioning the extensor mechanism. Often release of either longus or brevis will suffice rather than both (select depending on which seems tight)
	EDL tenotomy	Dorsal, proximal to MTPJ	Can be selectively released using a stab incision approximately 2 cm proximal to the MTPJ	Depends on other concurrent procedures to the toe	

(continued on next page)

Table 1
(continued)

Type	Description	Approach	Summary of Technique	Stabilization	Comments
					Also preferable to avoid release of either EDB or EDL in hammer toe as these naturally extend (correct) flexion deformity at level of PIPJ when closing P1 osteotomy for correction of MTPJ level deformity
MTPJ capsular release ± collateral release	Dorsal, at level of MTPJ	Incision made at level of MTPJ to right side (if right-handed). The Beaver Blade can then be introduced to the joint and the dorsal capsule released. If release of the collateral ligaments is required (eg, dorsal dislocation of MTPJ), then the blade can then be reintroduced (after partial reduction of the MTPJ afforded by the capsular release) and swept in a rotation either side of the MTPJ to release these	In the case of subluxation and dislocation at the level of the MTPJ, stabilization required; will depend on the resting stability of toe at the end of the surgery to achieve reduction	See algorithm for treatment of hammer toe (see **Fig. 11**).

| Bone surgery | P1 osteotomy for extension deformity of MTPJ (a bicortical osteotomy can be used to increase correction incorporating shortening) | Plantar, just distal to the MTPJ as located with the fingers of the NDH | The NDH stabilizes the toe (gripping the MTPJ between index finger dorsally and thumb on plantar aspect). The incision for the osteotomy is then made midline, just distal to the MTPJ on the plantar surface (distal to the surgeon's thumb on the plantar surface of the MTPJ). The 8-mm Shannon is then introduced via the portal and will abut the flexor sheath. The surgeon then steers the burr to the right side of the flexor sheath so that it lies against the bone of the proximal diaphyseal-metaphyseal junction of the P1. Leaving a dorsal bridge of cortex intact, the burr is then run at low speed and the osteotomy created by rotating the burr from right to left being careful not to translate the burr, which could place the flexor tendons at risk. | The osteotomy is closed in a plantar direction and is usually sufficiently stable that simple taping or strapping can be used to stabilize the osteotomy postoperatively | Used to correct extension deformity at the MTPJ level (see hammer toe algorithm, **Fig. 6A**). Plantar transtendinous approach and dorsal approach have also been described. Beware making the osteotomy more proximal than the diaphyseal-metaphyseal junction as this may risk injury to the flexor tendons where they are fixed in the A1 pulley or may result in an intra-articular fracture on attempting to close the osteotomy |
| | Straight P1 osteotomy for varus/valgus toe alignment correction | Midaxial or plantar depending on surgeon preference | For midaxial approach, the surgeon will approach from appropriate side of the toe, such that the osteotomy created will close and correct deformity in the direction required. The burr is introduced into the P1 at the proximal diaphyseal metaphyseal junction and swept in dorsal and plantar direction. | Taping usually sufficient | Elegant technique to correct varus/valgus deformity of the lesser toes (see **Fig. 6C**) |

(continued on next page)

Table 1
(continued)

Type	Description	Approach	Summary of Technique	Stabilization	Comments
	Oblique P1 osteotomy for varus/valgus toe alignment correction and shortening	Dorsomedial/ dorsolateral incision at distal P1 metaphyseal flare	The 8-mm Shannon burr is introduced into the P1 distal metaphyseal-diaphyseal junction (perpendicularly) and then rotated to the obliquity required in a proximal direction. The cut is then completed in 2 stages. An initial dorsal and plantar sweep of the burr will create the distal (near) half of the osteotomy. The burr is then advanced and the second proximal (far) half of the osteotomy completed. This osteotomy can be used to shorten the P1 and also correct supination/ pronation deformity as well as varus/valgus deformity present.	Taping usually sufficient	Very powerful technique for correction of severe deformity such as crossover second toe deformity (see **Fig. 6B**) Beware friable dorsal skin at entry point: wash out with saline to remove bone slurry and fine suture to close portal recommended Using a burr with longer cutting flutes is not recommended as may risk soft tissue injury
	P2 osteotomy (dorsal closing wedge)	Midaxial (right side of toe for right-handed surgeon) at mid P2 level	Via the midaxial incision, the 8-mm Shannon is inserted through both the near and far cortex. Raising the burr dorsally then completes the dorsal limb of the osteotomy. The plantar cortex can be thinned (but not completely cut) by lowering the burr in a plantar direction. The dorsal closing wedge osteotomy is then closed.	Often unstable and is best controlled by dorsal dermatodesis (excision of dorsal skin ellipse, which is then closed with fine nylon suture)	For correction of PIPJ level deformity Avoid trying to make the osteotomy closer to the PIPJ as this will often result in an intra-articular osteotomy (see **Fig. 6D**)

Condylectomy	Dorsolateral/dorsomedial distal to PIPJ	A straight periosteal elevator instrument is first introduced to create a working space up to the dorsal P1 prominence. Then the 8 mm Shannon burr is introduced to remove the P1 prominence. Chondral debris and slurry are then cleared by flushing with saline via the portal and rasping (MIS rasp instrument) via the portal.	Depends on other concurrent procedures; generally not performed in isolation	This is generally not required, and if considering, then probably wise to consider PIPJ fusion instead as PIPJ will be stiff after condylectomy
Excision of exostosis or bony prominence	Depends on position of prominence	Incision generally distal to prominence to avoid damage to portal while burring. Straight elevator to create working space and 8-mm Shannon burr to remove prominence.	None required	Useful for simple bony prominence removal
Joint surgery (fusion)	PIPJ fusion	Midaxial (right side of toe for right-handed surgeon) at level of PIPJ	The 8-mm Shannon burr is introduced into the joint and the 2 surfaces are prepared by directing pressure onto the P1 and P2 surfaces (assisted with the NDH applying the respective phalanges against the cutting burr). Chondral debris and slurry are then cleared by flushing with saline via the portal and rasping (MIS rasp instrument [Wright Medical USA]) via the portal.	K-wires give best stability (Redfern prefers 2 × 1-mm K-wires to control rotation and allow contouring of the toe with wires in situ; wires easily cut and bent flush over the tip of the toe)	Useful in severe PIPJ deformity (as with open PIPJ fusion)
	DIPJ fusion	Midaxial (right side of toe for right-handed surgeon) at level of DIPJ	The 3-mm Shannon burr is introduced into the joint and the 2 surfaces are prepared by directing pressure onto the P2 and P3 surfaces (assisted with the NDH applying the respective phalanges against the cutting burr). Chondral debris and slurry are then cleared by flushing with saline via the portal and rasping (MIS rasp instrument) via the portal.	K-wires or Steri-Strip over terminal phalanx/DIPJ	Useful in severe DIPJ deformity (as with open DIPJ fusion)

Abbreviation: MIS, minimally invasive surgery.

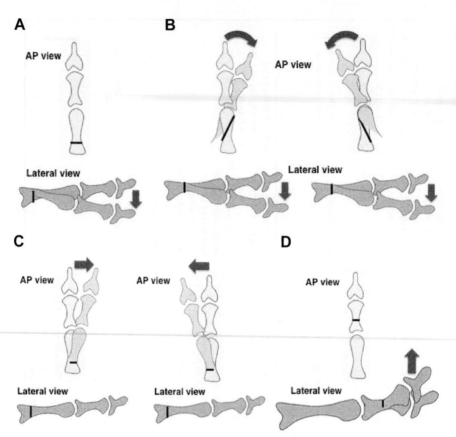

Fig. 6. (A) P1 unicortical plantar closing wedge osteotomy (dorsal cortex left intact). This can be used to correct sagittal plane deformity at MTPJ, and it can be made bicortical to increase power of correction in sagittal plane and shorten the toe. (B) P1 oblique bicortical osteotomy. This will shorten and correct varus or valgus, depending on the direction of the obliquity. It can also correct sagittal plane deformity (plantar flexion), if present. (C) P1 unicortical varus/valgus closing wedge osteotomy for correction of varus/valgus toe deformity. (D) P2 unicortical dorsal closing wedge osteotomy for correction of sagittal plane deformity at the PIPJ.

surgery), the gauze dressings are removed in favor of taping or commercially available toe alignment splints (once portal healed), which are applied to the toe to control its position for a further 3 to 4 weeks. Full weight-bearing in a stiff-soled postoperative shoe is recommended but with strict elevation for the 7 to 10 days after surgery.

The timing and frequency of further surgeon review during the first 6 weeks after surgery depends on the patient's ability to manage and reapply the taping/strapping. It is important that the surgeon ensures the taping/strapping is effective during the 6-week period following surgery in order to optimize the final result.

Example A

A 78-year-old man presented with painful valgus overriding deformity of his left third toe that was causing difficulty with footwear. Percutaneous second and third toe P1 oblique osteotomies were undertaken as shown in **Fig. 8**. The patient was able to return to ordinary footwear at 3 weeks after surgery.

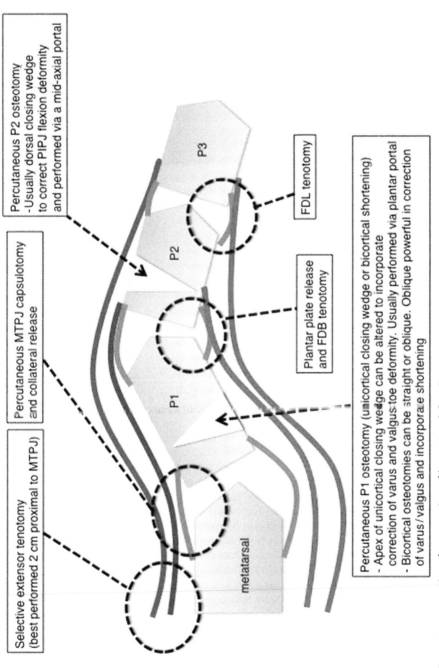

Fig. 7. Percutaneous options for correction of lesser toe deformity.

Percutaneous P2 osteotomy
-Usually dorsal closing wedge to correct PIPJ flexion deformity and performed via a mid-axial portal

Percutaneous MTPJ capsulotomy and collateral release

Selective extensor tenotomy (best performed 2 cm proximal to MTPJ)

FDL tenotomy

Plantar plate release and FDB tenotomy

P3

P2

P1

metatarsal

Percutaneous P1 osteotomy (unicortical closing wedge or bicortical shortening)
- Apex of unicortical closing wedge can be altered to incorporate correction of varus and valgus toe deformity. Usually performed via plantar portal
- Bicortical osteotomies can be straight or oblique. Oblique powerful in correction of varus/valgus and incorporate shortening

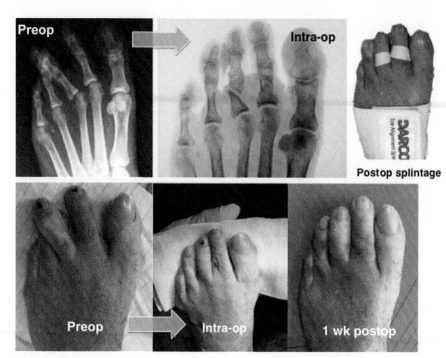

Fig. 8. Example A. Percutaneous second and third toe P1 oblique osteotomies to correct severe valgus deformities.

Hammer Toe Deformity

It is important to understand the etiology of hammer toes, and although attenuation or failure of the static stabilizers (including the plantar plate [PP]) may be important in the initiation of the deformity, it is the dynamic stabilizers (ie, flexors and extensors) that perpetuate the deformity. Although in the neutral/normal toe alignment situation, the flexors act as strong plantar flexors of the MTPJ, once the MTPJ is in dorsiflexion, they are weak flexors of the MTPJ (hence, weakness of paper pullout test) and relatively strong flexors of the interphalangeal joints. Similarly, the EDL is a strong extensor of the MTPJ in the hammer toe situation but relatively weak extensor of the interphalangeal joints. In other words, once the hammer toe has occurred, the flexors and extensors of the toe perpetuate the deformity (**Fig. 9**).

The key to reduction of the hammer toe (and maintenance of that reduction) is to balance the soft tissues; this can be achieved by neutralizing the toe position (with bone surgery predominantly), which in turn recruits the extensors and flexors of the toe to act in favor of maintaining the reduction and restoring toe function.

It is the authors' opinion that this approach negates the need for repair of the PP. In the recently published work of Nery and colleagues,[8] 60% of grade II PP lesions in their sample only had grade 1 instability and 45% of grade III PP lesions also only had grade 1 instability (grade 1 instability = laxity on drawer test of <50%). These figures do not seem to suggest strong correlation between the grade of PP rupture and the degree of clinical instability. Perhaps other stabilizers such as the collateral ligaments are more important.[9] The reported results are also of concern as to the effectiveness of repairing this damaged/pathologic tissue with high rates of persisting loss of ground touch (45% in grade 0, 50% in grade I and 62% in grade IV).

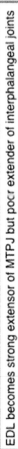
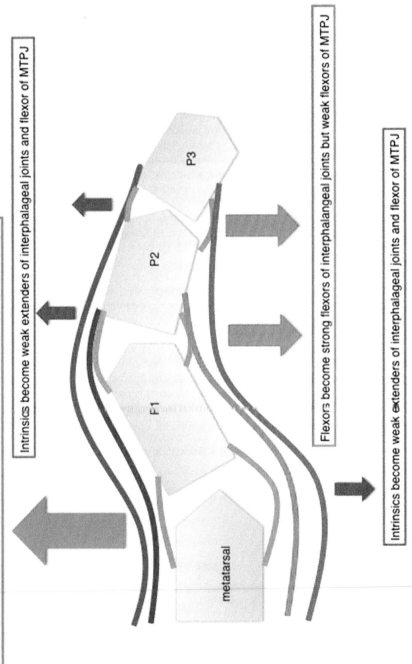

EDL becomes strong extensor of MTPJ but poor extender of interphalangeal joints

Intrinsics become weak extenders of interphalageal joints and flexor of MTPJ

Flexors become strong flexors of interphalangeal joints but weak flexors of MTPJ

Intrinsics become weak extenders of interphalageal joints and flexor of MTPJ

P3

P2

F1

metatarsal

Fig. 9. The dynamic stabilizers as deforming forces in the hammer toe.

Patients do not present complaining of a "plantar plate rupture" but do present with metatarsalgia and/or pain from the lesser toe deformity interfering with the upper of the toe box of their footwear. The key to success is to adequately correct the deformity *and* to address the etiology, whether that lies in the forefoot (eg, hallux valgus) or more proximally in the foot or calf (or both). In this way, the patient's complaints are adequately addressed and the risk of recurrence is minimized.

Although proximal phalanx osteotomies have been described with open techniques, they are difficult to stabilize and far more elegantly performed using percutaneous techniques. Percutaneous techniques allow for correction of both MTPJ level deformity (P1 osteotomy) and PIPJ level (P2 osteotomy) (**Fig. 10**).

Percutaneous techniques allow the surgeon to correct toe deformity in 3 planes by planning the position and obliquity of the osteotomy as well as determining whether unicortical or bicortical (incorporating shortening). Redfern's algorithm for the percutaneous correction of hammer toe deformities is outlined in **Fig. 11**.

It is the authors' preference to try and avoid division or lengthening of the flexors/extensors so as to avoid imbalance of the dynamic stabilizers; this is demonstrated by considering a flexible mild- to moderate-severity hammer toe. If a percutaneous P1 plantar closing wedge osteotomy is performed, then, as the osteotomy is closed in a plantar direction (see **Fig. 9**), the EDL extends the PIPJ, correcting deformity at that level. It will not do this if the surgeon has performed an extensor tenotomy.

With increasing severity of hammer toe, there is an increasing need to combine bone surgery with soft tissue surgery. In the case of MTPJ subluxation or dislocation, it is necessary to decompress the construct with a degree of P1 shortening via the osteotomy or PIPJ fusion (as would be the case with open techniques). There is therefore a need to include DMMOs in these circumstances.

If the MTPJ is subluxed or dislocated, then a percutaneous release of the dorsal capsule is first performed, allowing partial reduction of the joint. The Beaver Blade is then placed back into the MTPJ and the collateral ligaments are released, allowing further reduction. If necessary, an extensor tenotomy is performed at this stage (if the joint is still not reducible). If, after the above soft tissue releases, the joint remains irreducible, then a decision is made either to proceed to open reduction or to leave the joint dislocated (elderly/infirm or other specific circumstances). A good cosmetic result can still be obtained even with persisting dislocation at the MTPJ level and if the dislocation does not itself cause symptoms.

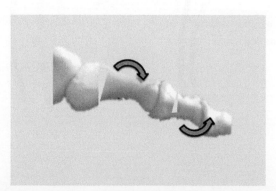

Fig. 10. P1 and P2 osteotomies for correction of sagittal plane deformity in hammer toe.

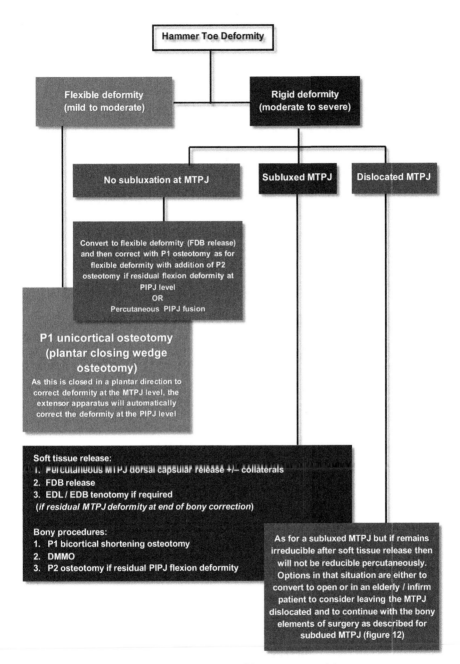

Fig. 11. Redfern algorithm for the treatment of hammer toes with percutaneous surgery.

Example B

An elderly patient presented with bilateral, severe crossover second toe, metatarsalgia, and associated hallux valgus (**Fig. 12**).

The surgical technique used for the right foot involved open fusion of the first MTPJ, and percutaneous dorsal capsular release of the second MTPJ, second MTPJ

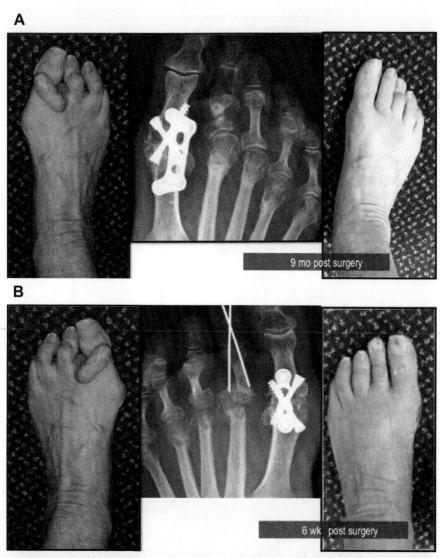

Fig. 12. Example B. Percutaneous treatment of dislocated crossover second toe. (*A*) Right foot. (*B*) Left foot.

collaterals, extensor tenotomy, and percutaneous shortening + rotating oblique P1 osteotomy, P2 osteotomy, and DMMOs M2-M4.

In the left foot, while the same surgical technique was used, the MTPJ was not reducible after the soft tissue surgery (as above), and a decision was made to leave the joint dislocated and correct the alignment of the toe as well as undertake DMMOs to treat her metatarsalgia adequately. The patient was equally happy with both feet at 9-month review after surgery and not aware of the residual dislocation of the second MTPJ in the left foot.

Complications

Thankfully, the risk of infection following these techniques is very low. Similarly, although some early sensory deficit in the operated toe is common in the first few weeks, this generally represents a neuropraxia and usually recovers after some weeks. The risk of vascular injury is very low if these techniques are carried out carefully (very low burr speeds), respecting the neurovascular bundles. Incomplete correction, recurrence, or even a new deformity can occur if the toe position is not well controlled in the first 6 weeks following the surgery.

Results

In 2009, Barbara Piclet[5] presented her results with percutaneous lesser toe correction at the 2nd Congress of Minimally Invasive Surgery in Murcia. The study reported the results of 112 feet that underwent second toe deformity correction involving FDB tenotomy, PIP release, and P1 osteotomy. Postoperative review took place at 6 and 36 months. She reported 97% patient satisfaction: 78% were assessed as good correction, and 19% were assessed as moderate but painless residual deformities. She observed recurrence in 3% of patients.

Piclet also presented a further study in April 2013 in Association Française de Chirurgie du Pied with a prospective series of 57 feet that had undergone percutaneous surgical correction of the second toe without any metatarsal surgery. She reported results of follow-up of more than 2 years (mean 30.7 months). In this study, she reported 90% patient satisfaction with the correction in all respects. Ninety-eight percent of patients were happy with the cosmetic result; 98% were happy with improvement in footwear comfort; 75% reported no footwear restriction, and 77% patients were pain free. Eight-eight percent of cases retained PIP flexibility; 86% had standing toe ground touch, and 86% had toe grasp present.

SUMMARY

Percutaneous techniques provide an alternative approach to lesser toe abnormality with far more versatility than traditional open techniques in terms of 3-dimensional correction while respecting basic surgical principles. As with all percutaneous techniques, it is vital the surgeon engage in cadaveric training from surgeons experienced in these techniques before introducing them into his or her clinical practice.

REFERENCES

1. Hofstaetter SG, Hofstaetter JG, Petroutsas A, et al. The Weil osteotomy: a seven-year follow-up. J Bone Joint Surg Br 2005;87(11):1507–11.
2. Beech I, Rees S, Tagoe M. A retrospective review of the Weil metatarsal osteotomy for lesser metatarsal deformities: an intermediate follow-up analysis. J Foot Ankle Surg 2005;44(5):358–64.
3. Maestro M, Besse JL, Ragusa M, et al. Forefoot morphotype study and planning method for forefoot osteotomy. Foot Ankle Clin 2003;8(4):695–710.
4. Khurna A, Kadamabande S, James S, et al. Weil osteotomy: assessment of medium term results and predictive factors in recurrent metatarsalgia. J Foot Ankle Surg 2011;17(3):150–7.
5. Redfern D, Vernois J, Legré BP. Percutaneous surgery of the forefoot. Clin Podiatr Med Surg 2015;32(3):291–332.

6. Henry J, Besse JL, Fessy MH, AFCP. Distal osteotomy of the lateral metatarsals: a series of 72 cases comparing the Weil osteotomy and the DMMO percutaneous osteotomy. Orthop Traumatol Surg Res 2011;97(6 Suppl):S57–65.

7. Haque S, Kakwani R, Chadwick C, et al. Outcome of minimally invasive distal metatarsal metaphyseal osteotomy (DMMO) for lesser toe metatarsalgia. Foot Ankle Int 2016;37(1):58–63.

8. Nery C, Coughlin MJ, Baumfeld D, et al. Prospective evaluation of protocol for surgical treatment of lesser MTPJ joint plantar plate tears. Foot Ankle Int 2015;35(9): 876–85.

9. Bhatia D, Myerson MS, Curtis MJ, et al. Anatomical restraints to dislocation of the second metatarsophalangeal joint and assessment of a repair technique. J Bone Joint Surg Am 1994;76(9):1371–5.

Minimally Invasive Osteotomies of the Calcaneus

Gregory P. Guyton, MD

KEYWORDS

- Minimally invasive • Calcaneus • Osteotomy • Burr • Dwyer • Medial displacement

KEY POINTS

- Minimally invasive calcaneal osteotomies have the same excellent healing potential and deformity correction as open techniques with potentially reduced pain.
- As long as appropriate anatomic landmarks are followed, the potential for neurologic injury is at least no worse than with open techniques; the potential for lateral calcaneal nerve injury may be reduced.
- A key benefit of the minimally invasive technique is the ability to place other incisions nearby, including those required for access to the peroneal tendons.
- Using a hinged jig to guide the osteotomy allows for readily reproducible cuts.
- Critical surgical steps include using a narrow spreader to ensure the release of the periosteum, evacuating the morselized bone fragments from the burr, and providing adequate fixation.

INTRODUCTION

Calcaneal osteotomies are powerful surgical tools to correct the weightbearing axis of the foot relative to the ankle and realign the pull of the Achilles tendon. They have utility both in the forms of medial and lateral displacement to address pes planus and pes cavus, respectively.

The Medializing Calcaneal Osteotomy for Pes Planus

The medializing calcaneal osteotomy was first described by Gleich[1] in 1893 to address pes planus deformity. Mechanically, its effect can be simplistically described as that of correcting a sagging tripod whose contact points are the heel, the first metatarsal head, and the fifth metatarsal head. By moving the heel medially, the sag is between the heel and first metatarsal is elevated. In 1973, the concept was subsequently applied by Koutsogiannis[2] to the correction of the flexible pediatric flatfoot with successful results.

Disclosure: Dr G.P. Guyton is a paid consultant for Tornier USA.
Department of Orthopaedic Surgery, MedStar Union Memorial Hospital, 3333 North Calvert Street, Baltimore, MD 21218, USA
E-mail address: gpguyton@gmail.com

Foot Ankle Clin N Am 21 (2016) 551–566
http://dx.doi.org/10.1016/j.fcl.2016.04.007
1083-7515/16/$ – see front matter © 2016 Elsevier Inc. All rights reserved.
foot.theclinics.com

The modern era of adult flatfoot reconstruction began with the recognition of the central role of posterior tibialis dysfunction in the genesis of the problem. Although repair of the posterior tibialis proved to be largely unsuccessful, in the 1980s Johnson and Strom,[3] and Mann and Thompson,[4] independently arrived at the concept of using the flexor digitorum longus tendon as a transfer to the navicular to replace its function. This led to significant pain relief but little correction of the deformity in many patients. Numerous investigators subsequently advocated applying Koutsogiannis'[2] experience with adolescents to adults by providing an element of deformity correction to the procedure with medial displacement calcaneal ostetotomy.[5,6]

The medial displacement calcaneal osteotomy has become a mainstay of the surgical correction of the adult flatfoot with associated hindfoot valgus,[6] although it is notable that the clinical results of flexor digitorum longus transfer alone in the early papers by Mann and Thompson,[4] and Johnson and Strom,[3] were remarkably good. No comparative psychometric results of the reconstructions with and without calcaneal osteotomy are extant. Nevertheless, the radiographic correction of numerous indices of foot alignment has been shown to be significant with the addition of a calcaneal osteotomy.

The Lateralizing Calcaneal Osteotomy for Pes Cavus

The lateralizing calcaneal osteotomy is a variation that may be used to address the hindfoot varus in pes cavus. The clinical problem is still regularly encountered today but it certainly does not dominate much of orthopedic practice as it did in the era of the poliomyelitis pandemic. Today most pes cavus corrections occur in the setting of idiopathic deformity or Charcot-Marie-Tooth disease.

A mobile subtalar joint usually allows sufficient eversion to prevent a fixed hindfoot varus from developing. In some cases of cavus foot deformity, correction of the medial column of the foot may be all that is required, usually by performing a dorsiflexion osteotomy of the first ray. Typically, the Coleman block test can be used to determine the level of flexibility of the subtalar joint. The hindfoot and lateral border of the foot are placed on a block of approximately 2 cm thickness, allowing the medial column to fall free. If the heel fails to move into a valgus alignment, the subtalar joint is immobile and a calcaneal osteotomy must be performed.

Several variations of the calcaneal osteotomy exist for the correction of hindfoot varus. Dwyer[7] originally described the removal of a wedge from the lateral wall of the bone while leaving the medial side intact as a periosteal hinge. Although this osteotomy was intrinsically stable and could be performed with minimal fixation, modern devices render this point moot. The use of a lateral shift allows for greater correction and adequate stability is easily achieved. Samilson[8] used a hinged crescentic osteotomy to displace the posterior tuberosity dorsally and reduce the calcaneal pitch. As an isolated procedure, this is rarely required today; extreme cases of high calcaneal pitch were most commonly encountered in specific patterns of polio. The variations of a lateral wedge, lateral shift, and vertical shift are not mutually exclusive and can readily be combined to deal with specific situations.

As a practical matter, most cases of hindfoot varus can be addressed without the addition of the resection of a bony wedge; they are, therefore, amenable to the same minimally invasive osteotomy techniques used for flatfoot.

Adjacent Incisions and Concomitant Procedures

Among the most compelling reasons for the use of the minimally invasive calcaneal osteotomy is to avoid affecting the incisions required for other elements of hindfoot reconstruction. This is particularly true in the case of the varus heel. Peroneal disease and chronic ankle instability are very commonly encountered with severe pes cavus.

Access to the peroneal area can usually be made through the same extensile lateral incision used for lateral ankle ligament reconstruction. However, adding a calcaneal osteotomy through the same incision is very difficult and requires retraction or extensive dissection of the sural nerve. Although no clear standards for incisional spacing on the lateral hindfoot exist, using a parallel oblique calcaneal incision near a very long peroneal incision raises real concerns for skin necrosis. A minimally invasive calcaneal osteotomy obviates these issues.

Risk to the Neurovascular Structures

A primary concern in any minimally invasive orthopedic surgery is that the primary goals be accomplished without additional risk to the neurovascular structures. Several specific nerves must be considered in the case of the calcaneal tuberosity.

The sural nerve

Traditional open techniques allow for direct visualization to avoid the sural nerve and mobilize it if necessary. Nevertheless, sural neuritis does occur as a complication of the procedure, potentially from overzealous retraction. To provide guidelines to avoid the sural nerve with the minimally invasive incision, Talusan and colleagues[9] described a safe zone based on intraoperative fluoroscopic landmarks. Their study used fine wires applied to the sural nerve along its passage over the calcaneus to localize the nerve radiographically. A perfect lateral image is obtained and a line from the plantar fascia origin to the posterosuperior apex of the calcaneus is drawn. A safe zone extending 11.2 plus or minus 2.7 mm can be defined anterior to this landmark line to avoid the sural nerve (**Fig. 1**). In practice, the incursions of the nerve into the safe zone occur at the

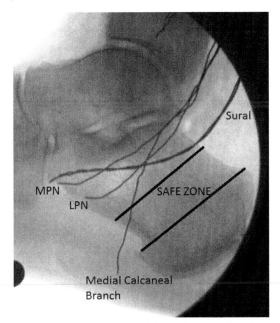

Fig. 1. The radiographic safe zone described by Talusan and colleagues[9] as shown in radiograph with the nerves outlined by fine wires. It provides a minimum of 2 mm of clearance from the main trunk of the sural nerve. MPN, medial plantar nerve; LPN, lateral plantar nerve. (*From* Talusan PG, Cata E, Tan EW, et al. Safe zone for neural structures in medial displacement calcaneal osteotomy: a cadaveric and radiographic investigation. Foot Ankle Int 2015;36:1495; with permission.)

superior aspect of the calcaneus; if incision placement is carefully limited to the center of the tuberosity, the anterior limit of this zone can be routinely used. Using these land-marks, no sural nerves were encroached on in 10 cadaveric specimens in a separate limb of the study by Talusan and colleagues[9] to validate the technique.

The medial and lateral plantar nerves
The placement of the osteotomy with respect to the medial and lateral plantar nerves is no different with the percutaneous technique than with the open technique. Exces-sive anterior placement may place these structures at risk on the medial side. As with the open technique, maintaining an osteotomy plane normal to the lateral wall of the calcaneus avoids this concern. The routine use of axial calcaneal fluoroscopy at the time of burr placement is recommended.

Bruce and colleagues[10] performed an MRI-based cadaveric study suggesting that the volume available for the tarsal tunnel is significantly reduced by lateralizing calcaneal osteotomies. They also noted that more anteriorly placed osteotomies put the medial neurovascular structures at greater risk. Only case-report and anecdotal evidence exist that medial and lateral plantar nerve entrapment occurs following the procedure; sys-temic evidence is not available. Whether clinically significant or not, the effect would not be expected to be different in magnitude with open versus percutaneous techniques.

Medial and lateral calcaneal branches
Smaller posteriorly directed nerves are routinely encountered passing from the sural nerve laterally and from the tibial branches medially to supply the posterior heel. The lateral nerves are particularly vulnerable and injury is common. They often pass directly across the incision for an open approach to the lateral calcaneus, and are either unrec-ognized or cut of necessity so that a sagittal saw can be positioned for the osteotomy.

The minimally invasive technique requires only small dissection of less than 1 cm through the most vulnerable zone for these sensory branches and essentially requires no retraction to accomplish the osteotomy. Paradoxically, it provides a potential element of safety for these small branches. In the validation arm of the study of Talusan and colleagues,[9] 1 of 10 specimens had a lateral calcaneal nerve injury with a minimally invasive technique compared with 3 of 10 with the open procedure.

INDICATIONS AND CONTRAINDICATIONS FOR THE MINIMALLY INVASIVE TECHNIQUE

The medial displacement calcaneal osteotomy can be safely performed in any context in which the open technique is also used. Lateralizing osteotomies are somewhat more difficult to displace, and the addition of a bony wedge resection to the procedure may be best done open (**Table 1**).

SURGICAL TECHNIQUE
Preoperative Planning

Calcaneal osteotomies are almost always performed in conjunction with additional procedures.

Table 1
Indications and contraindications for the minimally invasive technique

Indications	Contraindications
All standard indications for open procedures	Lateral wedge resection added to displacement for severe varus deformity
	Large dorsal displacement osteotomy for high calcaneal pitch

- The critical choice in pes planus reconstruction is to determine the order in which they are to be performed.
  - If the predominant deformity is abduction through the transverse tarsal joint, the Evans procedure should be performed first.
  - If hindfoot valgus predominates, the calcaneal osteotomy should be performed first.
  - If medial column instability predominates, a stabilizing procedure (first tarsometatarsal or naviculocuneiform fusion) should be performed first.
- The foot should be reassessed following the first procedure. The degree of correction may be surprisingly large, eliminating the need for additional procedures.
- In pes cavus reconstruction, a Coleman block test (or clinical assessment of subtalar mobility) will help determine whether a calcaneal osteotomy is necessary.

Patient Positioning

- A full lateral position is ideal if feasible.
- A removable bump under the ipsilateral hip allows the leg to be internally rotated.
- When possible, all lateral procedures can be performed first. The bump is then removed to allow access to the medial structures.

Surgical Approach

- A perfect lateral fluoroscopic image should be obtained.
  - Ideal overlap between the 2 arcs created by the medial and lateral shoulders of the talus should be obtained.
- The safe zone defined by Talusan and colleagues[9] is established by projecting anteriorly 11 mm from a line drawn between the posterosuperior apex of the calcaneus and the plantar fascia origin.
- The incision should be made directly in the middle of the tuberosity at the anterior edge of the safe zone. An 8 mm oblique incision is made parallel to the anticipated course of the osteotomy.
- Spreading dissection with a small hemostat parallel to the oblique incision (and the expected course of the sural nerve) is made to bone (**Fig. 2**).

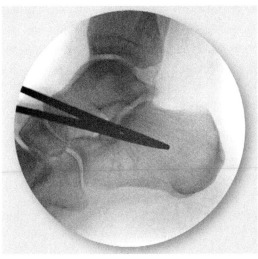

Fig. 2. A hemostat used to localize the incision location at the anterior margin of the safe zone on a perfect lateral radiograph. The center of the tuberosity is chosen.

- A narrow periosteal elevator (eg, a Joker, Freer, or Crego) is used to pass subperiosteally above and below the margins of the calcaneus along the expected course of the osteotomy.

SURGICAL PROCEDURE (JIG-ASSISTED TECHNIQUE)
Burr and Jig Placement

- A 2.5 or 3 mm Shannon burr is placed into the bone in a position normal to the lateral bone surface. The far medial cortex should be barely penetrated.
- Lateral and axial calcaneal images are checked to ensure appropriate placement.
  - On the lateral image, the burr should be exactly at the described position of the anterior margin of the safe zone.
  - On the axial image, the burr should be perpendicular to the long axis of the calcaneus.
  - Minor adjustments in calcaneal length can be made by slightly adjusting the angulation of the burr.
    - Anterior angulation will lead to greater foreshortening of the calcaneus if a medial displacement is performed.
    - Posterior angulation will lead to slight lengthening as a medial shift is performed. Although this will make up for the kerf of the burr cut, it may also make a medial shift more difficult to achieve.
  - The jig (Wright Medical, Memphis, TN) (**Fig. 3**) is now placed over the burr, taking care to ensure that the base of the jig is against the lateral side of the bone.
  - Using the same perfect lateral fluoroscopic view, the jig is rotated until the line of the osteotomy is visualized as just anterior to and parallel to the metal guide arc of the jig (**Fig. 4**).
    - When the desired oblique line of the osteotomy is obtained, 2 transfixing K-wires are placed through the jig into the calcaneus.
- Note that the jig is oriented with all its supporting structure to keep these wires in the posterior tuberosity and away from the sural nerve.

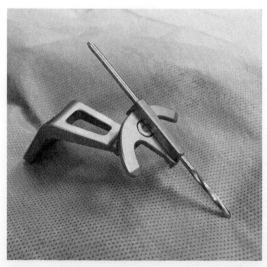

Fig. 3. A metal hinged jig created to guide a Shannon burr for calcaneal osteotomy.

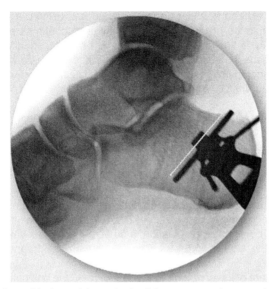

Fig. 4. The jig in place with the anticipated axis of the osteotomy just anterior to the guide arm.

Cutting the Osteotomy

- The Shannon burr is used in a sweeping motion to create the osteotomy. The jig is designed to allow the burr to rotate around a fixed point just above the near cortex of the bone (**Fig. 5**). Typically, a fan-shaped path through the cancellous bone is created first without penetrating the far cortex. This serves to further template the cutting through the harder medial cortical bone.
- In denser bone, typically in an adolescent, sweeping through the far cortex can be difficult. A series of small vertical penetrations can be made to fenestrate the path of the osteotomy. These can then be connected with a sweeping motion.
- The jig does not allow sufficient range of motion to allow the burr to reach the near (lateral) cortex. A shorter burr is recommended for greater control. The jig

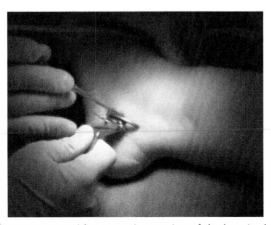

Fig. 5. Creating the osteotomy with a sweeping motion of the burr in the jig. An assistant stabilizes the jig in addition to the K-wire fixation into the calcaneus.

is then removed and the near cortex is penetrated using a freehand technique (**Fig. 6**). Completion of the cut can be difficult to confirm by tactile sensation alone; a change in the audible pitch of the burr may be equally informative.

- On occasion, the clearest evidence that the cut is complete will come from the lateral fluoroscopic image. The kerf of the burr passage is usually readily visible. If it disappears, the 2 fragments are now free and have collapsed against each other (**Fig. 7**).
- A narrow laminar spreader is now used to spread the fragments and aid in parting any remaining periosteal hinge.
- With the laminar spreader in place the osteotomy site should be deeply irrigated and evacuated of the morselized bone fragments (**Fig. 8**).

Shifting the Osteotomy

- The ankle should be plantarflexed to relax the Achilles tendon.
- For medializing osteotomies, a shift of 8 to 13 mm is typical. If adequate shift is not achieved by simple manipulation, a small periosteal elevator can be placed underneath the lateral cortex to lever the tuberosity fragment into position (**Fig. 9**).
- Lateral shifts are of lower magnitude, depending on the position of the cut. A shift of 7 to 10 mm is typical.
  - Other than inadequate release of the periosteum, the most common reason for difficulty in shifting the cut is an excessively posterior position, which allows for greater tethering of the posterior fragment by the plantar fascia (**Fig. 10**).

Fixation

- A 0.062 K-wire is used to provide axial temporary fixation once the initial shift has been applied (**Fig. 11**).
- In cases of a lateral shift, an axial screw is typically used.
  - The screw should be oriented normally to the osteotomy and headed for the denser subchondral bone underneath the subtalar joint.
  - The less dense bone in the empty triangle under the angle of Gissane provides less holding power. A screw oriented in this direction will provide less holding power and may have to be larger in diameter.

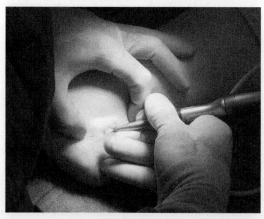

Fig. 6. Completion of the near cortices using a free-hand technique with the burr outside the jig.

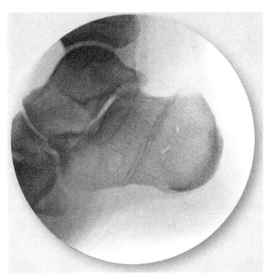

Fig. 7. Closure of the osteotomy indicates the fragments are free to move and that the cut is complete.

- The screw for a lateralizing osteotomy should be placed lateral to the midline so any compression achieved will tend to provide further lateralization of the heel pad.
- In patients with adequate bone quality, lower profile fixation options are possible to reduce the substantial risk of hardware pain. A single 4.5 mm headless screw is often sufficient.
- Screws or a percutaneous blade plate (Wright Medical, Memphis, TN) can be used for the medializing osteotomy. The blade plate provides very stable fixation while aiding in obtaining an adequate shift and avoiding the morbidity of an incision on the apex of the heel (**Box 1**).

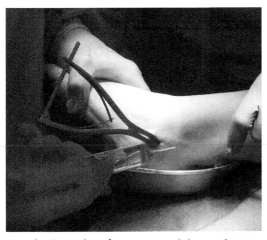

Fig. 8. A laminar spreader is used to free any remaining periosteum, and the marrow contents and bone fragments are evacuated via irrigation and suction.

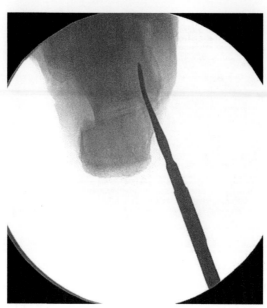

Fig. 9. A periosteal elevator is used to hinge under the lateral cortex and aid displacement if necessary.

COMPLICATIONS AND MANAGEMENT

Complications following the procedure are rare. Delayed would healing and drainage from the osteotomy site are most common. This is successfully managed with simple dry dressing changes and elevation as required. Patients should be made aware of the possibility that it may take up to 1 month for the wound to mature (**Box 2**).

POSTOPERATIVE CARE

- Calcaneal osteotomies typically take place as part of a complex of procedures for correction of the pes cavus or pes planus deformity. Other bony work, such as an Evans osteotomy or a midfoot fusion, typically requires 6 weeks of non-weightbearing and will determine the pace of rehabilitation.
- In the rare event that a calcaneal osteotomy is performed alone or in conjunction only with other soft tissue procedures, healing of the calcaneus proceeds rapidly enough that 4 weeks of nonweightbearing immobilization alone is sufficient.

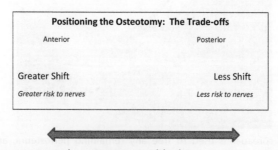

Fig. 10. Anterior versus posterior osteotomy positioning.

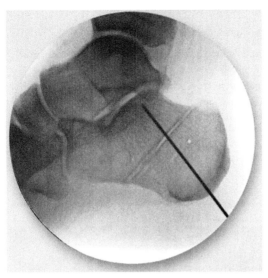

Fig. 11. A 0.062 K-wire is used for temporary fixation.

Box 1
Blade plate fixation of the percutaneous medializing calcaneal osteotomy

- Once adequate temporary fixation is achieved, make a temporary mark on the inserter arm to align with an 8 mm skin incision over the lateral heel approximately 2.5 cm posterior to the original osteotomy incision (**Fig. 12**).

- A periosteal elevator is used to tunnel between the 2 sites.

- Using the temporary mark as a guide, the blade plate is tunneled along the same path and driven into the proximal fragment (**Figs. 13–15**).

- A drill is now used through the cannulated set screw on the blade plate to drill through the locking hole in the proximal fragment. Sighting off the inserter arm, care must be taken to ensure the drill is aligned orthogonally with the plate in all axes (**Fig. 16**). Alternatively, a locking tower can be applied to the locking hole of the plate after the inserter is removed.

- The set screw holding the blade plate to the inserter is now released through the original incision. The inserter is rocked laterally to fully disengage it from the blade plate and removed.

- A locking screw is now placed.

- The drill guide for the compression screw is placed obliquely in the pocket of the plate aiming anteriorly and medially. Avoid excessive overpenetration of the far cortex because the drill path may head directly through the sustentaculum and toward the medial neurovascular bundle (**Fig. 17**).

- Undersize the pocket screw by at least 4 mm to avoid overpenetration medially. If an Evans osteotomy more anteriorly is contemplated, avoid a screw longer than 30 mm to stay away from the anterior process (see **Fig. 17**; **Fig. 18**). Usually the compression achieved in the softer cancellous bone is modest but the already placed blade plate and locking screw are adequate fixation alone in most patients.
  - Use fluoroscopy if necessary to ensure the screw is going into the pocket of the plate if there is any concern. If the screw misses the plate, it will easily penetrate into the soft cancellous bone of the cut edge of the osteotomy. This can be difficult to retrieve.

Box 2
Avoiding and managing wound healing complications

1. Irrigate if necessary during creation of the osteotomy. Substantial heat is generated particularly in high-quality bone.

2. Meticulously irrigate all marrow contents from the osteotomy once it is complete.

3. Use nylon instead of than absorbable sutures for closure of the osteotomy wound. They are less reactive and will provide holding power for longer if necessary.

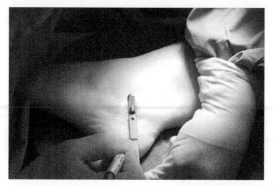

Fig. 12. A temporary mark is made on the inserter arm at the site of the posterolateral incision.

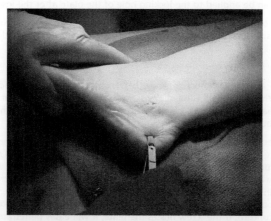

Fig. 13. The blade plate is tunneled along the lateral aspect of the bone and driven in place with a mallet.

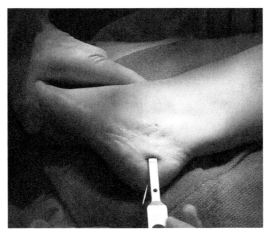

Fig. 14. The previous mark can be used to guide the depth of the insertion.

- The initial nonweightbearing period is followed by 4 weeks of ambulation in a CAM boot. During this time, physical therapy may be initiated, patients may sleep without the boot, and active motion is allowed.

OUTCOMES

Relatively few reports are available on the results of minimally invasive calcaneal osteotomies. In the largest series to date, Kendal and colleagues[11] reported a series of 31 cases over 6 years, along with a concurrent cohort of 50 open surgeries. The investigators reported a similar degree of calcaneal shift and overall excellent outcomes, although the single nonunion in the series occurred in the minimally invasive group. Sural nerve injury occurred in 6% of the open cohort versus none in the minimally invasive surgery (MIS) group. A lower rate of wound complications was reported in the MIS group versus the open group (6.45% vs 28%). Wound infection was also

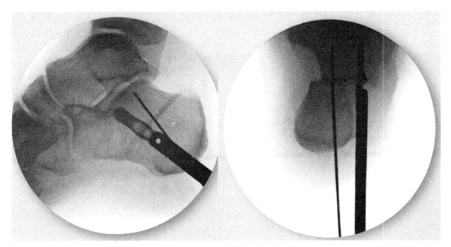

Fig. 15. Radiographs also guide the depth of the insertion (*left*) and ensure the blade plate is indeed underneath the lateral cortex (*right*).

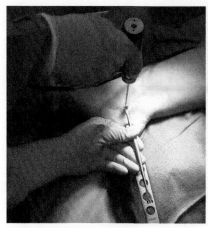
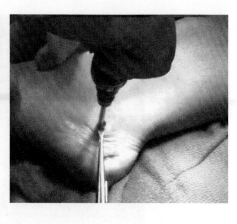

Fig. 16. The locking screw is drilled through the cannulated set screw (*left*) holding the blade plate to the inserter arm (*right*). An orthogonal position is required.

reported as lower in the MIS group (3% vs 20%). Inpatient hospital stays were shorter by an average of half a day. The outcomes generate some concerns, including the very high rate of wound complications with the open techniques, higher than those reported in previous series, and the potential for selection bias in this nonrandomized study. Additionally, pes planus correction is typically performed on an outpatient or 23-hour admission basis in North America; the data on inpatient stay may be difficult to interpret.

Kheir and colleagues[12] reported a series of 30 subjects from a sequential series performed by 2 surgeons. No nerve complications, wound complications, malunions, or nonunions were reported. No comparative open data were available.

The author's personal series includes 73 sequential cases performed by a single surgeon over 27 months, 48 of which were performed after development of the guiding jig. Only 1 open osteotomy was performed during the time of the series due to an intraoperative equipment failure. Ten cases were performed as lateralizing osteotomies in conjunction with pes cavus correction; the remaining 63 were performed as part of pes planus corrections. No cases of malunion or nonunion have occurred. Seven patients

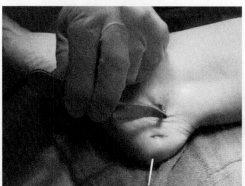
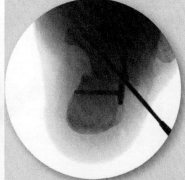

Fig. 17. The pocket screw is placed. The passage of the pocket screw often aims down the sustentaculum and toward the medial neurovascular bundle (*left*). Radiographic view (*right*).

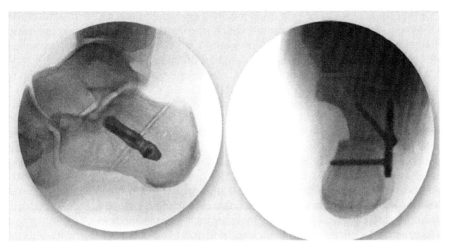

Fig. 18. The final placement of the blade plate encounters the harder subchondral bone beneath the subtalar joint and avoids the anterior process of the calcaneus. This avoids any interference with any potential Evans procedure. Lateral (*left*); axial/calcaneal (*right*).

experienced delayed wound healing, and 5 patients were placed on antibiotics and dressing changes. No return trips to the operating room for infection were required. Two plates were removed due to hardware pain.

These provide encouraging early data on the safety of the procedure. The surgical results clearly demonstrate equivalency with the open technique and suggest there may be potential advantages in wound healing, avoidance of nerve injury, and postoperative pain. Confirming superiority on the technical outcomes will likely require a randomized controlled trial of the 2 techniques. Pain relief is substantially more difficult to measure given the wide range of additional procedures typically performed in conjunction with calcaneal osteotomy.

SUMMARY

Minimally invasive calcaneal osteotomies offer the same excellent mechanical correction and reliable union rates as open techniques. It is clear that they are at least equivalent to open procedures with regard to safety and reliability. As long as appropriate anatomic landmarks are followed, the potential for neurologic injury is minimized. In fact, laboratory studies indicate that the potential for lateral calcaneal nerve injury may be reduced compared with the open procedure, and the only large comparative series of the MIS and open techniques indicated a lower incidence of sural nerve injury.

A key benefit of the minimally invasive technique is the ability to place other incisions nearby, including those required for access to the peroneal tendons. This is most beneficial in reconstruction of the cavus foot in which peroneal and lateral ankle ligament work are most commonly required.

Although freehand osteotomies can readily be performed, using a hinged jig to guide the osteotomy helps create readily reproducible cuts. Because of the relative distance from the adjacent joints, ease of fluoroscopic evaluation of the calcaneus, and ready potential to convert to an open procedure if necessary, the calcaneal osteotomy is a good candidate procedure for a surgeon gaining early experience with minimally invasive techniques.

Critical surgical steps include using a narrow spreader to ensure the release of the periosteum, evacuating the morselized bone fragments from the burr, and providing adequate fixation. The advantages of working on the well-vascularized calcaneus with its large surface area and rapid healing time apply as readily to the minimally invasive technique as to the open procedure. Weightbearing in cases without other bony procedures can be initiated 1 month postoperatively.

Because conformational surgery of the foot involves so many smaller procedures performed in conjunction with each other, the maximal benefits of minimally invasive techniques will not be realized until all components can be performed in a reliable fashion through percutaneous incisions. This ultimately includes the associated tendon reconstruction of either the peroneal or the posterior tibialis, lengthening osteotomies of the anterior process, midfoot osteotomies, and midfoot fusions. Attempts to measure reductions in postoperative pain or improvements in function will likely fall short as long as only the calcaneal osteotomy is altered in scope. Instead, converting the calcaneal osteotomy to a minimally invasive incision represents a first step toward a much more significant long-term goal of reducing the morbidity of these complex and continually challenging procedures.

REFERENCES

1. Gleich A. Beitrag zur operative plattfussbehandlung. Arch f. klin Chir 1893;46: 358–62.
2. Koutsogiannis E. Treatment of mobile flat foot by displacement osteotomy of the calcaneus. J Bone Joint Surg Br 1971;53:96–100.
3. Johnson KA, Strom DE. Tibialis posterior tendon dysfunction. Clin Orthop Relat Res 1989;239:196–206.
4. Mann RA, Thompson FM. Rupture of the posterior tibial tendon causing flat foot. Surgical treatment. J Bone Joint Surg Am 1985;67:556–61.
5. Guyton GP, Jeng C, Krieger LE, et al. Flexor digitorum longus transfer and medial displacement calcaneal osteotomy for posterior tibial tendon dysfunction: a middle-term follow-up. Foot Ankle Int 2001;22:627–32.
6. Myerson MS, Corrigan J, Thompson F, et al. Tendon transfer combined with calcaneal osteotomy for the treatment of posterior tibial tendon insufficiency: a radiological investigation. Foot Ankle Int 1995;16:712–8.
7. Dwyer FC. Osteotomy of the calcaneum for pes cavus. J Bone Joint Surg Br 1959;41:80–6.
8. Samilson RL. Crescentic ostetomy of the os calsis for calcaneocavus feet. In: Bateman JE, editor. Foot science. Philadelphia: Saunders; 1976. p. 18.
9. Talusan PG, Cata E, Tan EW, et al. Safe zone for neural structures in medial displacement calcaneal osteotomy: a cadaveric and radiographic investigation. Foot Ankle Int 2015;36:1493–8.
10. Bruce BG, Bariteau JT, Evangelista PE, et al. The effect of medial and lateral calcaneal osteotomies on the tarsal tunnel. Foot Ankle Int 2014;35:383–8.
11. Kendal AR, Khalid A, Ball T, et al. Complications of minimally invasive calcalneal osteotomy versus open osteotomy. Foot Ankle Int 2015;36:685–90.
12. Kheir E, Borse V, Sharpe J, et al. Medial displacement calcaneal osteotomy using minimally invasive technique. Foot Ankle Int 2015;36:248–52.

Minimally Invasive Arthrodesis of 1st Metatarsophalangeal Joint for Hallux Rigidus

A.H. Sott, FRCS (Tr&Orth)

KEYWORDS

- Hallux rigidus • Minimally invasive forefoot surgery • Arthrodesis
- Patient-reported outcomes

KEY POINTS

- Arthrodesis, or fusion of the 1st metatarsophalangeal joint (MTPJ), is considered the gold standard of surgical treatment of the very painful arthritic big toe joint.
- Several open, and few, minimally invasive/percutaneous techniques have been described in the literature, with comparable fusion rates of 80% to 94%.
- The surgical technique involves a high-speed wedge bur for joint preparation with compression screw fixation under fluoroscopic control.
- Postoperatively, patients mobilize immediately fully weight bearing in an adapted shoe with little swelling and virtually no wound complications.
- Clinical fusion rates at 6 weeks are more than 90%, with radiologic 4-corner cross-trabeculation visible at 1 year in more than 85%.

INTRODUCTION

Hallux rigidus was originally described by Cotterill in 1887[1] as degenerative disease of the 1st MTPJ with subsequent stiffness and clinical deformity. After hallux valgus it is the second most common pathology of the first ray. Patients present with stiffness and loss of function, ranging from inability to wear shoes due to osteophytes to often being unable to run or even walk without severe pain. Radiologic signs of severe osteoarthritis include joint space narrowing, cysts, sclerosis, and osteophyte formation. The age of presentation is widely variable; however, the mean age is in the fourth decade. A majority of cases are unilateral at initial presentation; however, development of bilateral disease is as high as 80% over 9 years[2] (**Fig. 1**).

The author has nothing to disclose.
Foot & Ankle Unit, Trauma & Orthopaedics, Epsom & St Helier University Hospitals NHS Trust, Wrythe Lane, London SM5 1AA, UK
E-mail address: Andrea.sott@esth.nhs.uk

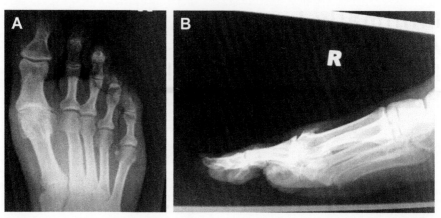

Fig. 1. (*A*) AP radiograph of arthritic painful 1st MTPJ/hallux rigidus. (*B*) Lateral radiographs of arthritic painful 1st MTPJ/hallux rigidus.

Surgical options to relieve the presenting severe pain and stiffness of advanced osteoarthritis include cheilectomy, distal metatarsal osteotomy, arthroplasty, and metatarsophalangeal arthrodesis. Choice of technique is based on patient-specific factors, such as the trade-off between mobility and pain relief. First MTPJ arthrodesis plays a significant role in the treatment of hallux rigidus and is considered the gold standard treatment in advanced (stage 4) disease. Several open and 2 percutaneous techniques have been described in the literature[3,4] using a variety of osteosynthesis techniques and surgical methods. Reported rates of clinical and radiologic fusion in the literature range from 80% to 100%.[5–7]

The primary determinants of outcome and satisfaction with MTPJ arthrodesis are thought to be the 3-D positioning of the arthrodesis, the method of joint surface preparation, and the choice of osteosynthesis. The consensus in the literature suggests fusion of the joint in a position of neutral rotation and some dorsiflexion with approximately 10° of valgus.[8–13] Preparation of the joint surfaces is achieved through reamers, burs, or a saw. The joint is prepared to 2 flat surfaces or to convex and concave surfaces. The latter is hypothesized to reduce the incidence of ray shortening.[4,9] Osteosynthesis is achieved by wiring, staples, screws, and low-profile plates. The author presents a percutaneous technique for 1st MTPJ arthrodesis using 2 compression screws with fluoroscopic control with description of the operative technique, outcome, and discussion. The primary indication for arthrodesis of the 1st MTPJ is degenerative joint disease or hallux rigidus—fusion presents the gold standard in definitive treatment of this painful disabling condition. The indications and contraindications do not differ from primary open arthrodesis (**Box 1**).

SURGICAL TECHNIQUE
Preoperative Planning

We obtain weight-bearing anteroposterior (AP) and lateral radiographs in patients who wish to proceed with 1st MTPJ arthrodesis for severe treatment-resistant arthritis after obtaining informed consent. Patients consent to the procedure of 1st MTPJ arthrodesis with the aim of a pain-free, stable, and functional big toe joint. Patients understand that a percutaneous procedure is planned but on occasion needs to be converted to open fusion. Patients are scored preoperatively using the Manchester-Oxford Foot Questionnaire (MOXFQ) and visual analog scale (VAS) scores and are

---

Box 1
Indications and contraindications for minimally invasive arthrodesis of the 1st metatarsophalangeal joint

Indications

- Painful osteoarthritis of 1st MTPJ
- Painful rheumatoid arthritis of 1st MTPJ
- Severe MTPJ deformity with cross-over first/second ray and ulcer formation

Contraindications

- Active infection
- Failed previous arthrodesis

---

informed about the need for follow-up scoring as well as auditing the outcomes and complications. All patients undergoing minimally invasive procedures are entered into a database and we recently also added in the EDQ-5-DL as an additional marker for patient-reported outcome and general well-being postsurgically.

Patient Anesthesia and Positioning

All patients are admitted as day cases and receive regional or general anesthesia with a preoperative ankle block and a single dose of intravenous antibiotic on induction; no tourniquet is used. Patients are placed supine with the foot extending beyond the end of the operating table to facilitate the use of sterile wrapped mini c-arm fluoroscopy (**Fig. 2**).

Approach

Under fluoroscopic control, the primary surgical portal is made medially at the MTPJ line as the main portal for bone surface preparation. A further portal is created laterally as necessary as well as proximally to remove any osteophytes (**Figs. 3–5**).

Procedure

This percutaneous, fluoroscopic-guided technique uses a high-speed water-cooled bur (Wright Medical) with a selection of burs and rasps to create the osteotomy. A mini C-arm image intensifier system is operated by the surgeon to provide fluoroscopic guidance. Several cannulated screw options are available; however, we use cannulated 4.3-mm variable pitch headless compression screws (Wright Medical).

Bone surface preparation is performed through the primary portal using tactile feedback and fluoroscopic control. The bur is used while applying longitudinal traction on the first ray, and 2 congruous surfaces are created removing any remaining diseased cartilage. A 14-gauge cannula is used from lateral to wash out the debris with physiologic saline. Bony preparation and washout are performed repeatedly, with the final washout omitted to leave some bone paste acting as autograft (**Figs. 6** and **7**).

Positioning of the hallux is critical for good patient outcome and is facilitated by the slight convex/concave joint surfaces. We chose a clinically neutral position that allows flat positioning of the hallux against a firm surface while allowing movement at the interphalangeal joint. Sagittal positioning is checked by the use of a flat support. The intended position is then held with crossing Kirschner wires as part of the cannulated screw fixation system. Fixation is achieved by two 4.0-mm compression cannulated screws and confirmed on fluoroscopy in 2 planes (**Fig. 8**).

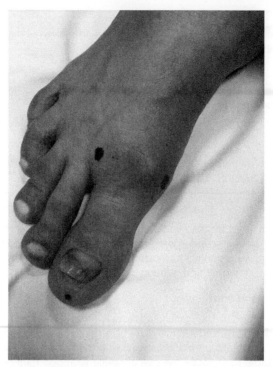

Fig. 2. Planned portals for MIS arthrodesis and joint preparation of 1st MTPJ.

Wounds are cleaned and closed with Steri-Strips and a compressive dressing is applied. A 1st MTPJ plaster splint and off-loader shoe are used to allow immediate postoperative heel weight-bearing mobilization (**Fig. 9**).

The average surgical time ranges from 25 to 40 minutes per case.

Patients are reviewed at 14 days for wound check and resplinting and then at 6 weeks with check radiographs. From this point, patients are advised to use rocker bottom shoes, such as Asics or MBT, provided there is evidence of clinical fusion

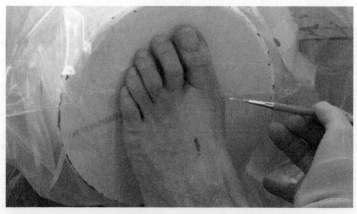

Fig. 3. Beaver Blade access to 1st MTPJ via medial image-guided approach.

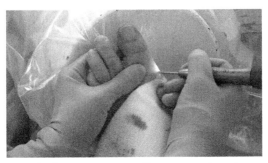

Fig. 4. Using 3.1-mm wedge bur to remove cartilage remnants and expose cancellous bone surfaces of 1st MTPJ under fluoroscopy.

and absence of pain. In cases of radiologic fusion that is not definite at 6 weeks, further follow-up is arranged.

Summary of Surgical Technique

1. Patient supine, sterile preparation, and draping of foot over distal edge of operating table with a mini c-arm ready to allow easy fluoroscopic control in AP and lateral planes.
2. If clinically indicated, perform cheilectomy via portal 1.5 cm proximal to MTPJ line (for technique see Razik A, Sott AH: Cheilectomy for Hallux Rigidus, in this issue).

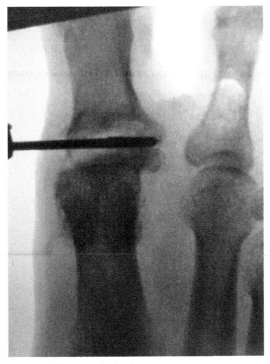

Fig. 5. Fluoroscopic image of intra-articular bur.

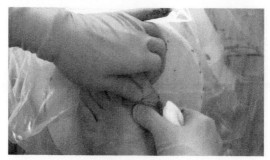

Fig. 6. Extrusion of bone and cartilage debris after bur preparation via medial portal.

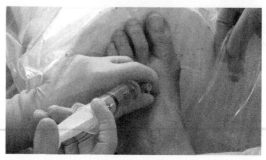

Fig. 7. Generous repeated irrigation to lavage bone debris during joint preparation.

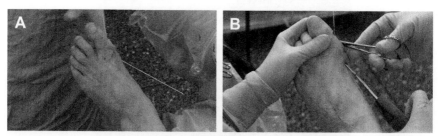

Fig. 8. (*A, B*) Fluoroscopic guided insertion of percutaneous compression screws to stabilize 1st MTPJ using guide wires and cannulated drills.

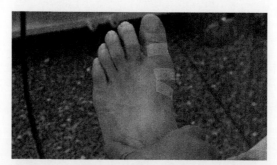

Fig. 9. Steri-Strip dressing to single-access portal and screw insertion sites after 1st MTPJ arthrodesis.

3. Use Beaver Blade to establish 2-mm medial portal under radiographic control to gain intra-articular access for 3.1-mm wedge bur (Wright Medical) to ream off articular cartilage remnants and expose cancellous bone surfaces.
4. While slightly distracting the joint, continue to establish congruent surfaces of M1 and P1, intermittently irrigating the joint with saline via lateral cannulated portal.
5. Align the 1st MTPJ in a neutral clinically plantigrade, rotation neutral, 5° valgus position, complementing the rest of the foot functionally, using a hard surface and holding this position with 1.6-mm Kirschner wire.
6. Check AP/lateral fluoroscopy for good bone contact and radiologic position and obtain fixation and compression with 2 crossed canulated 4.3-mm variable pitch headless compression screws under fluoroscopic control.
7. Use 1.2-cm Steri-Strips for the portals and add wool, POP gutter slab, and crepe to fit into a postsurgical heel weight-bearing shoe on crutches.

Pitfalls

Following training course, cadaver laboratory, and regular practice, the minimally invasive way of performing an arthrodesis of the 1st MTPJ is technically not too demanding; however, as with all surgical procedures, certain pitfalls need to be remembered (**Table 1**).

Surgeons need to be aware that in cases of soft bone or poor bone mass the bur pressure has to be particularly well controlled to avoid taking excess bone. As always, the option of converting to an open surgical procedure is available and patients should routinely be consented for both approaches. Further pitfalls and their management are found in **Table 1**.

POSTOPERATIVE CARE

Patients are discharged from the day case unit, with physiotherapy instructions on weight bearing in off-loader shoe on crutches and to allow elevation and rest. Patients are reviewed at 14 days for portal check and resplinting and then at 6 weeks with check radiographs. If there is clinical evidence of fusion (ie, a pain-free stiff joint on examination), patients are then advised to use rocker bottom shoes, such as Asics, and to avoid high impact for a further 6 weeks. If radiographs suggest delayed radiologic cross-trabeculation, further follow-up at 12 weeks and 6 months is arranged. As suggested by the National Institute for Health and Care Excellence, all patient data are collected for quality-control purposes in a dedicated database at our institution.

Table 1 Recommended management of pitfalls	
Pitfalls	**Management**
Sclerotic bone	Distract joint, alter the bur pressure against the surface in preparation. Observe expulsion of bone paste through portal on irrigation.
Soft bone/poor bone stock	Beware taking too much bone, convert to open procedure, and use plates or staples with bone graft.
Malpositioning of joint	Carefully align the foot clinically against rigid surface; clinically neutral dorsiflexion equals 10° radiologic dorsiflexion; the interphalangeal joint needs to be able to dorsiflex another 20°–30° off the rigid plate; check radiographs in true AP and lateral plates.

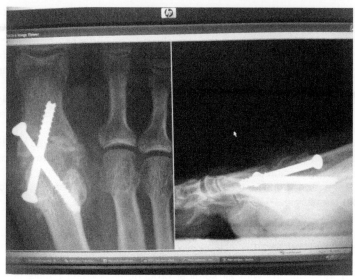

Fig. 10. Radiographs of 1st MTPJ arthrodesis at 6 weeks in outpatient clinic showing good alignment and radiologic fusion.

OUTCOMES

Few studies have been published about percutaneous or minimally invasive arthrodesis of the 1st MTPJ. Based on available evidence, clinical fusion is achieved in more than 90% of cases at approximately 8 to 12 weeks. A departmental 1-year review of cases showed an excellent percentage of patient satisfaction at 91%, with significant improvement in functional outcome scores (**Figs. 10** and **11**, **Table 2**).

SUMMARY

In summary, we believe that this technique provides a rapid uncomplicated percutaneous way to achieve clinically sound arthrodesis and a pain-free functional 1st MTPJ

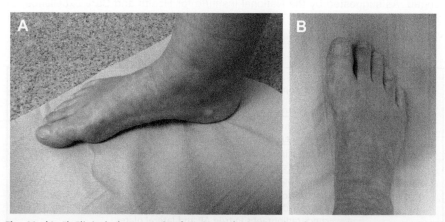

Fig. 11. (*A, B*) Clinical photograph of patient's foot 6 weeks after 1st MTPJ.

Table 2
Studies on percutaneous arthrodesis

	Follow-up	Fusion	Dorsiflexion Angle	Outcome	Revision
Bauer et al,[3] 2010 N = 32	18 m	31/32	21°	AOFAS pre 36 AOFAS post 80	Not stated
Fanous et al,[4] 2014 N = 26	3–20 m	Clin 23/26	14°	MOXFQ pre 32 MOXFQ post 18 VAS	3/26
Sott, 2015 Departmental audit data N = 18	12–24 m	Clin 16/18 Radiograph 12/18	12°	MOXFQ pre 34 MOXFQ post 19 VAS 91% very satisfied	0/18

with excellent clinical fusion rates and superb patient-reported outcome. In experienced hands, the procedure is simple, fast, and reproducible. Radiographic control allows surgeons to check positioning and fixation intraoperatively to obtain optimal fusion position for postoperative function. Postoperative recovery is uncomplicated and fast and patients generally return to trainer shoes at 6 weeks. We currently use percutaneous arthrodesis for all suitable cases and advocate this procedure to all foot and ankle surgeons after appropriate training.

REFERENCES

1. Cotterill JM. Stiffness of the great toe in adolescents. Br Med J 1887;1(1378): 1158.
2. Coughlin MJ, Shurnas PS. Hallux rigidus: demographics, etiology, and radiographic assessment. Foot Ankle Int 2003;24(10):731–43.
3. Bauer T, Lortat-Jacob A, Hardy P. First metatarsophalangeal joint percutaneous arthrodesis. Orthop Traumatol Surg Res 2010;96(5):567–73.
4. Fanous R, Ridgers S, Sott AH. Minimally invasive arthrodesis of the first metatarsophalangel joint for hallux rigidus. Foot Ankle Surg 2014;20(3):170–3.
5. Yee G, Lau J. Current concepts review: hallux rigidus. Foot Ankle Int 2008;29(6): 637–46.
6. Coughlin MJ, Shurnas PS. Hallux rigidus. Grading and long-term results of operative treatment. J Bone Joint Surg Am 2003;85-A(11):2072–88.
7. Groulier P, Curvale G, Piclet-Legre B, et al. Arthrodesis of the first metatarsophalangeal joint. Rev Chir Orthop Reparatrice Appar Mot 1994;80(5):436–44 [in French].
8. Kelikian AS. Technical considerations in hallux metatarsalphalangeal arthrodesis. Foot Ankle Clin 2005;10(1):167–90.
9. Curtis MJ, Myerson M, Jinnah RH, et al. Arthrodesis of the first metatarsophalangeal joint: a biomechanical study of internal fixation techniques. Foot Ankle 1993; 14(7):395–9.
10. Rongstad KM, Miller GJ, Vander Griend RA, et al. A biomechanical comparison of four fixation methods of first metatarsophalangeal joint arthrodesis. Foot Ankle Int 1994;15(8):415–9.

11. Harper MC. Positioning of the hallux for first metatarsophalangeal joint arthrodesis. Foot Ankle Int 1997;18(12):827.
12. Womack JW, Ishikawa SN. First metatarsophalangeal arthrodesis. Foot Ankle Clin 2009;14(1):43–50.
13. Goucher NR, Coughlin MJ. Hallux metatarsophalangeal joint arthrodesis using dome-shaped reamers and dorsal plate fixation: a prospective study. Foot Ankle Int 2006;27(11):869–76.

Percutaneous Pediatric Foot and Ankle Surgery

Michael G. Uglow, MBBS(Lond), FRCS (Tr&Orth)

KEYWORDS

- Minimally invasive surgery • Percutaneous foot surgery • Foot osteotomy
- Foot deformity correction • Cooled side-cutting burr • Pediatric foot • Child's foot

KEY POINTS

- Percutaneous techniques reduce wound problems by leaving minimal scar lengths, and require limited soft tissue dissection; bleeding and swelling associated with foot osteotomies are less likely to cause problems with percutaneous wounds.
- The cancellous bones of the child's foot cut easily with a new cooled side-cutting burr and healing times do not seem to be delayed with 6 weeks in the distal tibia being typical.
- Proper assessment and rebalancing of deforming forces is essential for prevention of recurrent deformities and tendon transfers must be performed where appropriate through standard open incisions in conjunction with minimal access wounds for bony correction.
- The percutaneous approach is ideal where scarring pre-exists from earlier surgery or such cases as burns where traditional open wounds are hazardous.

INTRODUCTION

The surgical correction of foot deformities in adults and children has changed notably over the last few decades with increasing knowledge of surgical outcomes coupled with technological advancements with the equipment available to surgeons. In adult practice perhaps the starkest example is from Charnley open arthrodesis through a transverse incision cutting all structures between the skin and joint[1] when compared with the contemporary arthroscopic arthrodesis with percutaneous screw fixation leaving minimal scarring.[2]

In children's practice the last two decades have seen a complete change in ethos in managing clubfeet from open surgical release to closed serial casting with the addition of a percutaneous Achilles tenotomy in the majority. This method has seen a reduction in rates of surgery from 80% to less than 5%, the latter mostly being attributed to atypical and syndromic cases.[3] A range of other foot deformities can be approached with similar ethos and this article explores the use of minimal-access surgery in correcting these problems.

The author has nothing to disclose.
Department of Paediatric Orthopaedics, University Hospital Southampton, Mailpoint 044, Tremona Road, Southampton SO16 6YD, UK
E-mail address: Mike.Uglow@uhs.nhs.uk

Foot Ankle Clin N Am 21 (2016) 577–594
http://dx.doi.org/10.1016/j.fcl.2016.04.005
1083-7515/16/$ – see front matter © 2016 Elsevier Inc. All rights reserved.

Minimally invasive surgery has been developed in foot and ankle surgery in the adult, particularly of the forefoot, using a cooled side-cutting burr (**Fig. 1**).[4] The author has found appropriate uses of this burr in cutting children's bones with very good effect. The results of femoral and tibial osteotomies in children have been presented previously[5] and in this article techniques for percutaneous osteotomies in children's foot practice are discussed. The use of the burr has been studied in adult cadaveric feet and found not to be injurious to the surrounding soft tissues.[6]

The purpose of foot surgery is to correct deformities and to rebalance the deforming forces that drive the abnormalities. If these principles are not followed then the deformity remains uncorrected or easily recurs. Open surgery is as much a part of this process as percutaneous surgery and the principles that are followed are to minimize the size of wounds where appropriate but make every step necessary to ensure correction and prevention of recurrence. Minimizing the incisions can reduce some of the complications (**Box 1**) and improve the cosmetic result of surgery.

CLINICAL ASSESSMENT

As with all deformity correction the surgeon has to assess the whole child but especially the entire lower limb and the foot's relationship to it, and the individual components of the foot. This article cannot do justice to the full assessment of the lower limb and foot in children but the reader is referred to the seminal work published by Mosca[7] for a full and thorough account: examination of the spine to establish if the pelvis is level, alignment of the lower limb (longitudinal and rotational), alignment of the hindfoot to the lower limb, alignment of the midfoot to the hindfoot, and alignment of the

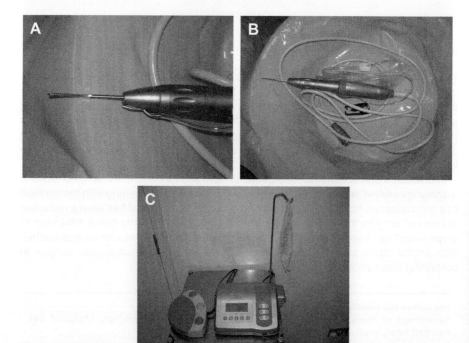

Fig. 1. Photographs of the equipment required to cut a percutaneous osteotomy with the burr. (*A*) The 2 mm × 20 mm side-cutting burr mounted in its handpiece. (*B*) The handset and burr with lead and tubing. (*C*) The control unit and foot pedal.

Box 1
Issues that are seen in open surgery

- Wound healing
- Bleeding
- Swelling
- Infection
- Neurovascular injury
- Scarring
- Scar contracture

---

forefoot to the midfoot. The essential aims of treatment in children are to establish lower limbs of equal length by maturity, longitudinal and rotational limb alignment within normal limits, a plantigrade painless foot by skeletal maturity, and a functional foot and lower limb.

DEFORMITIES THAT ARE CORRECTED USING PERCUTANEOUS METHODS
Rotational Malalignment of the Tibia: Rotation Osteotomy of the Tibia

Indications/contraindications
Internal and external tibial torsion are corrected using a supramalleolar osteotomy of the tibia (**Fig. 2**). Internal torsion is more common and less well tolerated than external torsion and is the deformity most commonly corrected. With an internal rotation deformity the hindfoot tends to inversion, which locks the foot during the stance phase of gait. Increased loading patterns are seen on the lateral border of the foot and particularly over the prominent fifth metatarsal base, which can result in pain. The subtalar complex and the ankle can be painful as can the knee with increasing degrees of rotation.

It is not uncommon to see children between the ages of 3 and 10 years with a negative foot progression angle. The whole limb must be examined and associated femoral anteversion is the most common cause but several cases present with either internal tibial torsion or a malrotation at the subtalar joint. The latter may be caused by an incompletely corrected hindfoot following clubfoot casting or by relapse. The first

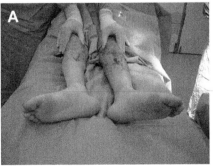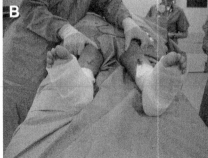

Fig. 2. Correction of external tibial rotation using a supramalleolar osteotomy. (*A*) Preoperative picture showing marked external rotation tibial deformity with some asymmetry. (*B*) Postoperative film showing symmetric correction.

option is to perform repeat casting using Ponseti principles but if repeat serial casting fails to reduce the subtalar joint the internal rotation deformity is corrected at the supramalleolar level.

This is a technically straightforward procedure with few risks and excellent outcome compared with trying to correct the deformity at the level of the pathology. It is technically more demanding to use an extra-articular osteotomy or a soft tissue release through the subtalar joint. The latter is associated with higher relapse rates and pain after the age of 4 years, although one would not choose to intervene with a tibial osteotomy until the potential for natural correction with growth has had time to have an effect if any.[8] The tibial osteotomy is therefore not usually performed before 6 years and preferably not until 9 or 10 years.

Surgical technique

Preoperative Planning
- Assess degree of internal or external rotation to correct from gait and clinical examination.
- In unilateral deformity the aim is to correct to match the unaffected side.
- Plain radiograph in two planes to ensure no longitudinal deformity exists.

Preparation and Patient Positioning
- General anesthesia plus
- Regional anesthesia
  ○ Using popliteal block for unilateral cases
  ○ Using caudal or epidural anesthesia for bilateral cases
- Supine on radiolucent operating table.
- Thigh tourniquet (with or without sandbag beneath to control position of foot).
- Skin preparation from above the knee to the toes so that correct rotation is assessed.

Surgical procedure

- Image intensifier in position from side of table.
- Mark the tibial physis with a skin marker.
- Mark the proposed site of osteotomy approximately 5 cm above the physis
- Make a 5-mm vertical incision over the mid fibula at this level (ie, anterior to posterior).
- Insert the first gently curved periosteal elevator and free the periosteum around the anterior and posterior fibula.
- Insert the second highly curved periosteal elevator around the fibula in both directions to free the periosteum circumferentially.
- Make a 5-mm vertical incision in the skin over the medial face of the tibia at the level of the proposed osteotomy.
- Use blunt dissection to reach the periosteum, avoiding the long saphenous vein and saphenous nerve.
- Use both periosteal elevators, as described for the fibula, to sequentially free the periosteum around the entire circumference of the tibia
- Insert a 2.0-mm K-wire through the medial malleolus aiming for the lateral tibial cortex at a point several centimeters proximal to the proposed osteotomy site. Leave the wire distal to the proposed site of osteotomy.
- Insert a second 2.0-mm K-wire into the lateral aspect of the distal tibial metaphysis just proximal to the physis, aiming for the posteromedial tibial cortex several centimeters proximal to the proposed osteotomy site, again leaving the

wire distal to the osteotomy site. Aiming this wire posteriorly avoids having both holding wires in the coronal plane (**Fig. 3**).

- Insert 2 mm × 1.6 mm short K-wires in the sagittal plane anteriorly, with one either side of the proposed osteotomy.
- Using the 2.0 mm × 13 mm side-cutting burr with a speed setting of 200 rpm and initial torque of 50 Nm, make a pilot hole through the fibula under image intensifier guidance.
- Using a gentle up and down rotating motion keeping the burr in the transverse plane, bring the burr to the anterior cortex of the fibula, followed by the posterior cortex. If resistance is felt, the machine automatically stops and the burr must be gently freed to allow it to start rotating again. If this occurs easily, the torque can be increased to a maximum of 80 Nm.
- The image intensifier is used to ensure completion of the osteotomy has occurred.
- The tibia is then osteotomized with the 2 mm × 20 mm burr using the same principle technique as described for the fibula. Care must be taken to ensure the "far cortex" is cut, which is at the furthest point from the entry hole at the posterolateral aspect of the tibia and is the hardest part to reach. Care is also required when exiting the posteromedial cortex and completing the medial cortex of the tibia. The burr is held in a vertical position at this point and the neurovascular bundle is protected by the posterior tibialis sheath. The burr must be kept in the transverse anatomic plane to ensure the osteotomy is in the plane of the joint.
- Once the osteotomy is completed the distal tibia is then rotated externally using the marking 1.6-mm anterior K-wires as a visual guide until the desired correction is achieved.
- The assistant then holds the distal tibia and foot in the corrected position while the surgeon advances the 2.0-mm K-wires across the osteotomy and into the respective opposite cortices.

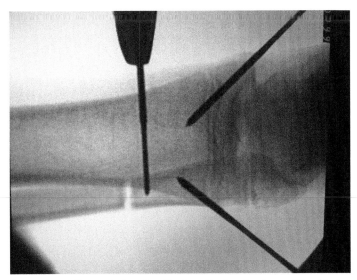

Fig. 3. Perioperative radiograph showing the two K-wires in situ and the fibula osteotomy already cut. The burr has been drilled through the tibia and is ready to cut the osteotomy in the plane of the joint.

- The image intensifier is used in the anteroposterior (AP) and lateral planes to ensure that the longitudinal alignment remains unaffected and the bone surfaces are opposed.
- The marking wires are removed.
- The wounds are lavaged to remove bone swarf from the skin but not from around the osteotomy, which aids union.
- Gauze is wrapped around the wires and then a well-padded cast is applied to below the knee with the toes exposed in the usual way.

Postoperative care

- The patient is managed routinely with leg elevation for a week and then allowed to mobilize non–weight bearing on crutches.
- The wires are removed, usually under general anesthesia at 6 weeks postoperatively and a radiograph taken.
- Typically a further cast is applied and the patient allowed to bear weight for a further 2 to 4 weeks depending on their age and the degree of healing seen on radiographs.

The appearance of the minimal scarring that can be expected is shown in **Fig. 4**.

Complications and management

- Failure to ensure that the burr remains in the transverse plane leads to an oblique osteotomy and angulation occurs together with the rotational correction.
- The aim is to align the second metatarsal with the midpoint of the patella or the tibial tubercle, if the latter is not laterally positioned. The marking K-wires ensure that the correction occurs at the osteotomy and that spurious correction does not occur by inadvertently rotating the tibia at the knee.
- Displacement at the osteotomy site can occur if the patient bears weight earlier than permitted and if the wires cross at the osteotomy site.
- In older patients the crossed wire technique becomes less reliable and this technique is sufficient up to the age of approximately 12 years. Thereafter, stability is conferred by using a plate and screws and as such there is no advantage to using the percutaneous burr technique in this age group.

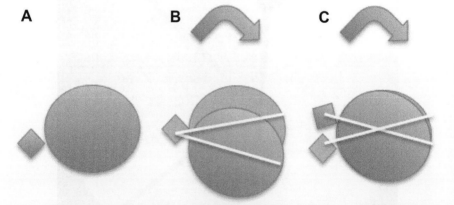

Fig. 4. Schematic showing the influence of the fibula to a tibial osteotomy. (*A*) The level of a left tibial osteotomy. (*B*) Without fibula osteotomy rotation occurs around the center of the fibula and posterior displacement and varus is produced in the tibia. (*C*) With fibula osteotomy allows ideal rotation around the center of the tibia.

Outcomes

The results were assessed in the first 20 tibial osteotomies performed,[5] which showed correction of the deformities in all cases. No wound infections were seen and all osteotomies were firm clinically and looked united at the 6-week check radiograph. The potential concern about heat generation and possible delay in union was not observed in these cases.

Discussion points

- The fibula must be osteotomized when performing a tibial rotation osteotomy for three reasons (see **Fig. 4**).
  - The center of rotation needs to be in the central axis of the tibia
  - The point of rotation becomes the axis of the fibula if it is not cut
  - A fibula osteotomy shortens the fibula the same amount as the tibia and prevents a varus deformity, albeit a small one.
- Alternative techniques are described to osteotomize the tibia, which include
  - Drill and osteotome
  - Gigli saw
  - Power saw

The drill and osteotome technique is popular because it is considered low energy. Some surgeons prefer this technique because the interdigitations of the cut osteotomy interlock and confer stability. The author's preference is to have two smooth surfaces, which allows accurate correction of the deformity, whereas interdigitation may give larger increments of rotation than desired.

The Gigli saw technique requires four incisions and may be difficult to maintain the saw within the transverse plane during cutting. For pure rotational correction the burr gives a secure way of maintaining this plane. The scarring following a burr percutaneous osteotomy is minimal (**Fig. 5**).

The power saw is a useful technique and quite straightforward. It is unlikely to create a problem of healing within the metaphyseal bone but does require a larger incision to perform. Healing following tibial osteotomy with a burr has not proved problematic (**Fig. 6**).

Malalignment of the Heel: Translation Osteotomy of the Os Calcis

For correction of excessive valgus or varus the tuberosity of the os calcis can be osteotomized and translated in either direction. The most common deformity is a

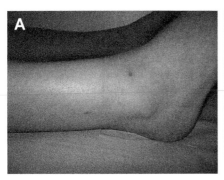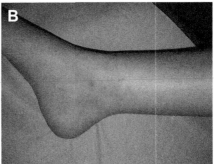

Fig. 5. The typical scars seen following a percutaneous osteotomy of the distal tibia. (*A*) The lateral scars and (*B*) the medial scars.

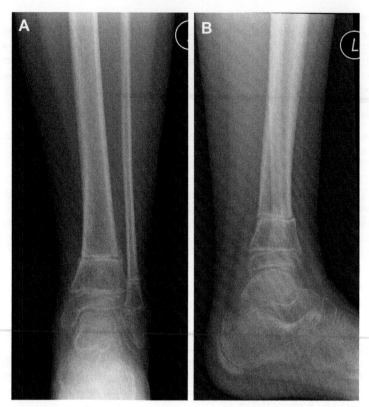

Fig. 6. Postoperative radiographs at 6 weeks after percutaneous tibial osteotomy. (*A*) AP view showing good alignment and healing. Note the wire tracks that cross at a site distant to the osteotomy. (*B*) Lateral view showing good alignment and good healing.

valgus malalignment that often coincides with a correctable flat foot pattern: the flexible pes planovalgus foot. If the subtalar complex and particularly the talonavicular joint are mobile then a lateral column-lengthening procedure with insertion of a cuneiform-shaped bone graft is the best option as advocated by Mosca.[9] This is not a procedure that can be performed percutaneously.

The lateral column-lengthening depends on the talonavicular joint being mobile allowing the mid and forefoot to rotate around a centre of rotation of angulation (CORA) in the talar neck.[10] For feet that have a fixed hindfoot deformity and when the talonavicular joint is stiff and does not allow correction, the malalignment is corrected by shifting the tuberosity. The most commonly used method is a straight oblique osteotomy through the body of the os calcis. Alternatives include a chevron-shaped osteotomy, which confers a greater inherent degree of stability at the cut osteotomy. A direct incision or extended lateral approach with elevation of the lateral flap can be used but this osteotomy lends itself to a percutaneous technique.

Indications

- Fixed hindfoot valgus
- Fixed hindfoot varus

Surgical technique

Preoperative Planning
- Assessment of amount of malalignment clinically.
- Assessment of degree of correctability of deformity and therefore suitability of tuberosity transfer.
- Radiographic assessment using Cobey or Saltzman view radiographs.

Preparation and Patient Positioning
- Lateral position on side with operating limb uppermost.
- Body supports to hold patient, vacuum bag device useful to aid repositioning perioperatively for the correction of other deformities, tendon transfers, and so forth.
- Check that leg can be rotated through 90° to allow AP view using image intensifier. If not, intensifier positioned to allow rotation of C-arm to obtain the AP view.
- Thigh tourniquet and skin preparation to expose the whole of the lower limb from the knee to allow proper assessment of correction.

Surgical approach

- With a straight metal edge and using the image intensifier, mark a straight line with a skin marker at the desired level for the osteotomy, about midway along the body of the os calcis.
- Mark the superior and inferior borders of the bone.
- Make a 5-mm incision in the middle of the premarked line through the skin only.
- Use blunt dissection to reach the periosteum, avoiding the sural nerve.
- Insert a small retractor into the wound; the assistant needs to hold this toward the dorsal aspect of the foot to protect the sural nerve until the cutting flutes are buried in the bone.
- Insert a 2 mm × 20 mm burr in patients younger than 10 years and a 3 mm × 20 mm burr for older patients, ensuring that the x-ray beam is perpendicular to the bone. It is best to align the limb horizontally on a support or by elevating the foot of the tale if adjustable.
- Keeping the burr vertical, advance like a drill through the lateral cortex and advance to the inner aspect of the medial cortex. A gentle bouncing technique gives good feel of contact with the harder cortical bone. Advance until the burr just penetrates the medial cortex.
- Remove the handpiece from the burr and check with the image that the burr is correctly positioned and correctly aligned. Reattach the handpiece.
- Keeping the burr upright, angulate the burr to cut the os calcis in line with the skin mark. It is preferable to keep moving to maintain the same plane but intermittently image is required to ensure that the burr does not stray from the chosen line of cut.
- Start with cutting a slot in the lateral cortex to give the burr some freedom and then advance along the medial cortex. The superomedial and inferomedial corners are the hardest to reach.
- Continue the osteotomy through the superior and inferior borders of the bone and then complete the lateral cortex.
- The burr is withdrawn and completion confirmed with the image intensifier (**Fig. 7**).
- The tuberosity is grasped and then moved in the chosen direction, medial or lateral depending on the direction of correction. If the bone does not move easily, a bony or soft tissue tether needs to be identified and released. This is done by inserting a flat instrument (McDonald or Freer elevator) into the osteotomy and feeling around the edges.

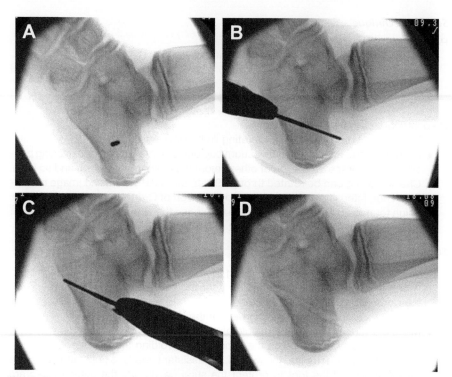

Fig. 7. Percutaneous translational osteotomy of the os calcis. (*A*) Burr drilled through the center of the line of osteotomy. (*B*) Cutting through the dorsal cortex. (*C*) Cutting through the plantar cortex. (*D*) Completed oblique osteotomy with wide surface area of contact.

- Once free, the bone is easily displaced. Inspection along the line of the lower leg guides how much to shift the bone. The same flat instrument can be inserted into the wound to ensure that one can feel a definite step between the adjacent cortical surfaces to ensure displacement is as desired.
- The tuberosity is moved easily when the ankle is in plantar flexion and once the desired correction has been achieved the ankle is dorsiflexed to tension the soft tissues and lock the tuberosity until fixation is in place. Correction of alignment should be undertaken in consideration of the correct relationship of the hindfoot axis to the long axis of the tibia as described by Paley.[11]
- For younger children the use of two smooth wires of 2.0 mm to 2.5 mm passed from the posterior surface of the heel across the osteotomy into the body of the os calcis is perfectly adequate fixation. Once the apophysis of the heel is beginning to close, a 6.5-mm cannulated screw is used (Headless Compression Screw, Synthes, West Chester, PA) is preferred because the screw can be buried.
- The skin is lavaged to remove swarf, which may cause skin irritation.
- Other procedures can then be performed as indicated and once complete the limb is placed in a well-padded below-the-knee split cast or back slab.

Postoperative care

- The patient is managed routinely with leg elevation for a week and then allowed to mobilize non–weight bearing on crutches.
- If a back slab is used this is changed for a full cast 10 to 14 days postoperatively.

- The wires are removed under general anesthesia at 6 weeks postoperatively.
- A fiberglass cast is applied for 6 weeks and the patient allowed to weight bear during this time.
- The cast is removed at 12 weeks postoperatively and a radiograph taken to ensure healing.

Complications and management

- The sural nerve is at risk during this procedure.
  - Blunt dissection beneath the skin and using a retractor during use of the burr prevents this.
- Position of the osteotomy incorrect.
  - If too close to the apophysis the tuberosity fragment may get tethered by the attachment of the plantar fascia and not displace easily.
  - Fixation may be less secure if the thickness of the fragment is too thin.
  - If too close to the subtalar joint the joint could be encroached and the available space for fixation reduced.
- The neurovascular bundle is at risk if the burr penetrates too far through the medial cortex and if the osteotomy is placed closer to the subtalar joint than is needed.
- The flexor hallucis longus tendon is at risk beneath the sustentaculum if the osteotomy is placed too close to the subtalar joint.
- If the osteotomy is not performed keeping the burr perpendicular to the long axis of the os calcis the osteotomy will be made in an oblique plane such that the tuberosity lengthens or shortens when translated. If the plane is forcing lengthening then the soft tissues become tighter and prevent adequate translation of the tuberosity fragment.
  - Correct orientation of the burr prevents this.
  - In older children, the 3-mm burr gives more freedom to move the tuberosity because more bone has been removed during cutting.

Discussion points

The fixed varus hindfoot can be corrected very well using the Dwyer lateral closing wedge osteotomy[12] and is best performed through an open approach. This is performed percutaneously using a wedge burr but is technically challenging to complete evenly across the entire width of the bone surface and the translation osteotomy is technically easier and more predictable. If the desired correction is more than about 15 mm or if the soft tissue envelope on the medial side is likely to tether the neurovascular bundle then an open traditional Dwyer procedure is a better option.

Midfoot Deformities

Indications

Several deformities in the midfoot are amenable to percutaneous osteotomy. Several techniques are available in the literature and include drill and osteotome, osteotome alone, Gigli saw, and power saw. The Gigli saw technique was described by Paley and Tetsworth[13] and has recently been presented with clinical outcomes for complex midfoot deformity by Lamm and colleagues.[14] Passage of the saw is controlled by using two parallel wires along the osteotomy corridor avoiding divergence and to contain the saw within bone throughout.

The cancellous nature of the foot bones makes them ideal for using the cooled side-cutting burr. The Gigli saw requires the use of four incisions, whereas the burr uses only two 5-mm incisions. The burr cuts through bone easily, especially in children, and does not cut the soft tissues surrounding the bone making it safe to use. The author has used the device in the following situations:

- Cuboid recession ± soft tissue medial release for adductus
- Cuboid recession and cuneiform osteotomy for fixed adductus in older child
- Closing flexion osteotomy of cuneiform for planus deformity
- Closing extension osteotomy of cuneiform for modest cavus
- Opening extension osteotomy of cuneiform for more severe cavus
- Rotation osteotomy of entire midfoot

The exact location of the osteotomy is determined by the deformity to be corrected. The midfoot has several options for siting an osteotomy, which include anterior os calcis to talar neck, anterior os calcis to navicular, cuboid to navicular, and cuboid to cuneiform (**Fig. 8**). Anatomically the talar neck and anterior os calcis are in the hindfoot but for certain complex deformities the midfoot and forefoot rotation is better corrected at a more proximal level.

Surgical technique
Preoperative Planning

- Assessment of deformity in relation to hindfoot.
- Consideration of three planes of deformity.
  - Supination/pronation
  - Plantaris/extension
  - Adduction/abduction
- Weight-bearing radiographs in AP, lateral, and oblique planes to assess ideal osteotomy corridor.

Preparation and Patient Positioning

- Patient is positioned supine with the leg prepared to the knee to allow accurate assessment of correction.
- A sandbag placed under the tourniquet aids rotation of the limb for ideal placement of the foot.
- A support to go under the distal lower leg above the ankle is helpful to lift the foot for ease of access.

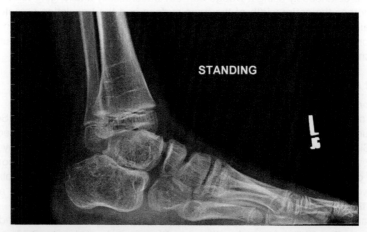

Fig. 8. Lateral radiograph of the foot demonstrating the cuboid-navicular and cuboid-cuneiform corridors for midfoot osteotomy.

Surgical approach

- The image intensifier is used to define the anatomy and skin marks placed to mark the osteotomy (the description assumes the cuneiform cuboid corridor is to be used) (**Figs. 9** and **10**).
- A line drawn against a straight edge serves as a guide during cutting to maintain the correct line of cutting.
- A 5-mm incision is placed in the skin adjacent to the center of the medial cuneiform on its medial surface.
- The soft tissues are cleared with blunt dissection.
- The curved periosteal elevators are used to clear the soft tissue from around the cuneiforms on the dorsal and plantar surfaces. The tibialis anterior tendon courses obliquely across the cuneiform as it heads toward its attachment on the first metatarsal and needs to be displaced inferiorly.
- Unlike cutting a long bone or the os calcis, the periosteum of the cuneiforms is not lifted from the cortical layer because one is not able to strip through the capsule to the intermediate and lateral bones. The plane is therefore extraperiosteal.
- Insert the 2 mm × 20 mm burr into the center of the cuneiform and drill across into the lateral cuneiform under image guidance using the skin marker as a visual guide.
- Move the burr dorsally and plantarly to complete the osteotomy. The periosteal elevator is inserted to ensure that the periosteal layer is separated. The long plantar ligament may need to be incised using a long handle knife.
- The procedure is then repeated from the lateral side of the foot through the cuboid.

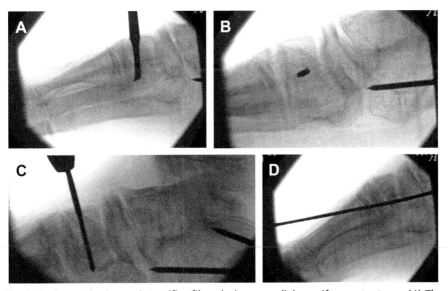

Fig. 9. Perioperative image intensifier films during a medial cuneiform osteotomy. (*A*) The periosteal elevator clearing the soft tissues around the site of osteotomy cut. (*B*) The burr bit is in the center of the bone before cutting. (*C*) Burr sweeping to the inferior cortex keeping in line with the joint surfaces. (*D*) Flexion of the first ray and the correction maintained with a K-wire. By preserving the dorsal cortex and taking increasing amounts of bone from the plantar aspect a wedge shape is removed to allow plantar flexion.

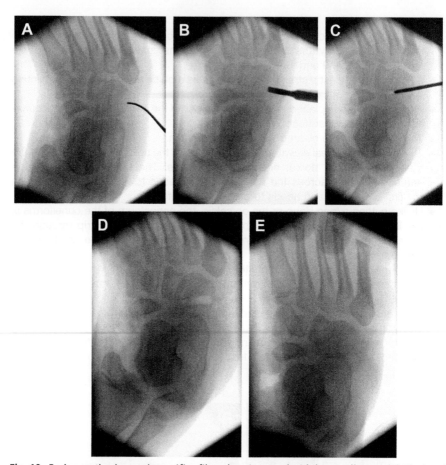

Fig. 10. Perioperative image intensifier films showing a cuboid decancellation. (*A*) The level of osteotomy is marked using a metal instrument. (*B*) Soft tissues are cleared with a periosteal elevator. (*C*) The 3-mm wedge burr is used to create an ever-increasing wedge-shaped slot in the cuboid. (*D*) Completed cavity in the cuboid is clearly shown. (*E*) Closure of the cuboid allows correction of the forefoot. In this case open reduction of the talonavicular joint was also performed. The air is seen in the medial tissues at surgery.

- If rotation is required, the forefoot is corrected to the desired position and then fixed with two smooth 1.6-mm or 2.0-mm K-wires depending on the size of the child.
- If correcting adduction deformity in the younger child between approximately 5 and 8 years the wedge burr is used to decancellate the cuboid. The initial osteotomy cut with the 2-mm Shannon burr is then opened using the wedge burr (see **Fig. 10**).

Postoperative care

- A below-the-knee back slab is applied or a split cast depending on preference.
- The limb is elevated for the first week and the child is kept non–weight bearing for 6 weeks.
- The cast is changed at 2 weeks to apply a full cast and the wires removed at 6 weeks postsurgery.
- A full weight-bearing cast is then applied for a further 6 weeks.

Considerations in the midfoot

Correction of adductus of the midfoot and forefoot is achieved in several ways. **Fig. 11** highlights the different methods and the implications particularly for the soft tissue envelope on the medial side. If one attempts to open the medial cuneiform only then the forefoot is not corrected, only the first metatarsal. Flexion and extension are corrected in the first ray by osteotomizing the medial cuneiform only but adduction requires division of all three of the cuneiforms. If one opens from the medial side to gain full correction the skin medially is lengthened too much so for larger corrections a combination of closing wedge in the cuboid and opening wedge in the cuneiforms gives a powerful correction with less lengthening and subsequent tension of the medial soft tissue envelope.[15,16] In older children transferring a wedge of bone to the medial side gives better results and as such open surgery gives better results than a percutaneous procedure.

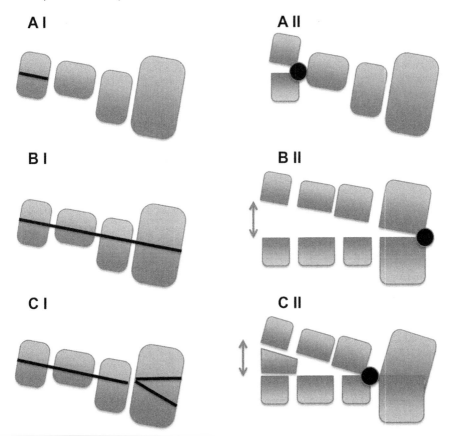

Fig. 11. Schematic showing the different outcomes of osteotomy cuts in the midfoot for correcting adductus. *Black lines* indicate osteotomy cut, *black circles* indicate point of rotation. (*A*) Osteotomy through the medial cuneiform only (*i*). Limited correction of adductus because only the first ray can be moved (*ii*). (*B*) Complete midfoot osteotomy (*i*). Excellent correction of adductus but significant lengthening can occur on the medial aspect causing increased soft tissue tension (*ii*). (*C*) Wedge resection of the cuboid and complete cuneiform osteotomy (*i*). Excellent correction of adductus occurs with less medial lengthening (*ii*). The point of rotation is at the lateral edge of the cuboid and the wedge of bone from the cuboid is used in the medial gap to maintain correction.

When correcting the flexible flat foot with a calcaneal lengthening osteotomy, there may be a fixed forefoot supination deformity. This deformity may be exaggerated by the lengthening and a medial cuneiform closing wedge osteotomy is performed to correct this. A 3-mm wedge burr is used percutaneously and the correction held with a K-wire or Steinmann pin to avoid adding an open procedure. This is an example where a combination of open and closed techniques are used, ensuring that the principles of full correction are followed but achieved with the minimal skin exposure possible.

An example of where a closed procedure is tried first but then subsequently an open soft tissue release is needed is demonstrated in **Fig. 12**. The adductus deformity is corrected using the percutaneous burr method but correction of the bone is seen to result in persistent varus of the hallux because of a short and tight abductor hallucis muscle. This needed open release of the medial soft tissues to achieve satisfactory correction.

COMPLEX FOOT DEFORMITIES AND GRADUAL CORRECTION WITH CIRCULAR FRAMES

For patients who have more complex deformities including equinus, varus, or where the heel is short and elevated, the posterior tuberosity is gradually corrected into an improved position using a circular frame and callotasis as described originally by Ilizarov and presented in the English literature by Grant and colleagues[17] and explained in detail by Kirienko and coworkers.[18] The osteotomy may have to be placed more distally to give a larger tuberosity fragment to ensure adequate fixation for the frame. The use of the burr is a real advantage in these cases to avoid having larger wounds present with the associated risks of swelling caused by more soft tissue dissection. Many of these more complex feet will have had surgery previously and a percutaneous procedure gives real advantage over open surgery and soft tissue dissection.[19]

Most surgeons have patients from the pre-Ponseti era but have seen a dramatic reduction in cases with scars from previous surgery as a result of the widespread

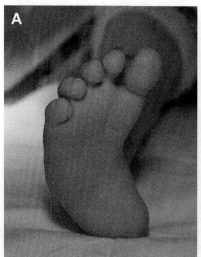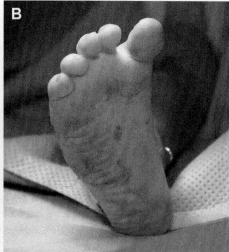

Fig. 12. Metatarsus adductus corrected by a percutaneous cuboid recession in a 4-year-old child. (*A*) Obvious curved convex lateral border of the foot with adductus of the forefoot. (*B*) After cuboid recession performed percutaneously showing good correction of the forefoot but persistent varus of the hallux. An open soft tissue release medially was performed.

> **Box 2**
> **Some diagnoses associated with stiff and complex foot**
>
> - Myelodysplasia
> - Diastematomyelia
> - Freeman-Sheldon syndrome
> - Diastrophic dysplasia
> - Arthrogryposis multiplex congenita

adoption of the Ponseti method.[20] For those who treat complex foot disorders in children with syndromes giving severe stiff feet (**Box 2**), surgical intervention is more than likely to be required at some stage during childhood. These feet often present a significant challenge to treat effectively and percutaneous techniques add to the range of options to minimize open wound exposure to reduce scarring.

SUMMARY

Percutaneous techniques for foot surgery have been described previously, commonly involving using a drill and osteotome and the Gigli flexible saw. The author has presented some examples of using a newer cooled side-cutting burr popularized in adult surgery for performing minimally invasive surgical techniques most notably of the forefoot and os calcis. The bones of the child's foot seem suited to being cut with the burr and correction of deformity using osteotomies cut in this way is performed through minimal skin access. The same principles of deformity assessment apply to any correction technique and most importantly the soft tissue deforming forces need to be rebalanced to prevent recurrences. Where necessary it is still necessary to perform open surgery for soft tissue release and tendon transfers but the addition of osteotomies with percutaneous access minimizes the soft tissue dissection that is needed with a corresponding reduction in wound size.

REFERENCES

1. Charnley J. Compression arthrodesis of the ankle & shoulder. J Bone Joint Surg Br 1951;33B:180–91.
2. Glick JM, Morgan CD, Myerson MS, et al. Ankle arthrodesis using an arthroscopic method: long term follow up of 34 cases. Arthroscopy 1996;12:428–34.
3. Morcuende JA, Dolan LA, Dietz FR, et al. Radical reduction in the rate of extensive corrective surgery for clubfoot using the Ponseti method. Pediatrics 2004; 113(2):376–80.
4. Vernois J, Redfern D. Percutaneous Chevron; the union of classic stable fixed approach and percutaneous technique. Fuß Sprunggelenk 2013;11(2):70–5.
5. Uglow MG. Percutaneous osteotomies of the femur and tibia using a cooled side cutting burr. Bone Joint J. Orthopaedic Proceedings 2014;96B(Supp 1):16.
6. Dhukaram V, Chapman A, Upadhyay P. Minimally invasive forefoot surgery: a cadaveric study. Foot Ankle Int 2012;33(12):1139–44.
7. Mosca VS. Principles and management of pediatric foot & ankle deformities and malformations. Philadelphia: Wolters Kluwer; 2014. p. 17–38.

8. Staheli L. Rotational problems in children. J Bone Joint Surg Am 1993;75A(6): 939–49.
9. Mosca VS. Calcaneal lengthening for valgus deformity of the hindfoot. Results in children who had severe, symptomatic flatfoot and skewfoot. J Bone Joint Surg Am 1995;77:500–12.
10. Mosca VS. Principles and management of pediatric foot & ankle deformities and malformations. Philadelphia: Wolters Kluwer; 2014. p. 222.
11. Paley D. Principles of deformity correction. Berlin Heidelberg: Springer-Verlag; 2002. p. 572.
12. Dwyer FC. Osteotomy of the calcaneum for pes cavus. J Bone Joint Surg Br 1959;41B(1):80–6.
13. Paley D, Tetsworth K. Percutaneous osteotomies: osteotome and Gigli saw techniques. Orthop Clin North Am 1991;22:613–24.
14. Lamm BM, Gourdine-Shaw MC, Thabet AM, et al. Distraction osteogenesis for complex foot deformities: gigli saw midfoot osteotomy with external fixation. J Foot Ankle Surg 2014;53:567–76.
15. Pohl M, Nicol RO. Transcuneiform and opening wedge medial cuneiform osteotomy with closing wedge cuboid osteotomy in relapsed clubfoot. J Pediatr Orthop 2003;23(1):70–3.
16. Lourenco AF, Dias LS, Zoellick DM, et al. Treatment of residual adduction deformity in clubfoot: the double osteotomy. J Pediatr Orthop 2001;21(6):713–8.
17. Grant AD, Atar D, Lehman WB. The Ilizarov technique in correction of complex foot deformities. Clin Orthop 1992;280:94–103.
18. Kirienko A, Villa A, Calhoun J. Ilizarov technique for complex foot and ankle deformities. New York: Marcel Dekker Inc; 2004. p. 8–16.
19. Uglow MG. Unpublished work, Podium presentation No 222 at The Combined Orthopaedic Meeting of the English Speaking World. Cape Town, 11th-15th April, 2016.
20. Ponseti IV. Treatment of congenital club foot. J Bone Joint Surg Am 1992;74: 448–54.

Neuropathic Minimally Invasive Surgeries (NEMESIS):
Percutaneous Diabetic Foot Surgery and Reconstruction

Roslyn J. Miller, FRCS (Tr&Orth)[a,b,]*

KEYWORDS

- Diabetes • Minimally invasive surgery • Charcot neuroarthropathy
- Charcot arthropathy • Neuropathic osteoarthropathy • Diabetic ulcer

KEY POINTS

- Neuropathic minimally invasive surgeries (NEMISIS) may offer potentially better surgical outcomes than traditional open surgical correction.
- The surgery is dependent on access to good multidisciplinary clinical working to ensure the best outcomes and improve the quality and duration of life of the diabetic patient with foot abnormality.
- NEMISIS may facilitate earlier stabilization and therefore shorten the treatment period and reduce the risk of amputation in this challenging patient group.

INTRODUCTION: NATURE OF THE PROBLEM
Global Impact of Diabetes

Every 6 seconds a person dies from diabetes.[1] Indeed, the mortality from diabetic foot ulceration is greater than that from some common cancers such as prostate and breast cancer, with 50% dying within 5 years.[2]

It is in North Africa, the Middle East, and South East Asia where the greatest impact is felt.[3] In global terms, the most significant impact of increasing prevalence is seen in the Middle Eastern countries of Saudi Arabia, Qatar, Bahrain, Kuwait, and the United Arab Emirates, of whom a significant number of patients remain undiagnosed.[3]

In England and Wales, the number of people diagnosed with diabetes has increased by approximately 53% between 2006 and 2013.[1]

Dr R. J. Miller is a Consultant for Wright Medical, Memphis, Tennessee.
[a] Department of Orthopaedics, Hairmyres Hospital, East Kilbride, Lanarkshire, UK; [b] The London Orthopaedic Clinic, London, UK
* Department of Orthopaedics, Hairmyres Hospital, East Kilbride, Lanarkshire, UK.
E-mail address: rosmiller@doctors.org.uk

Foot Ankle Clin N Am 21 (2016) 595–627
http://dx.doi.org/10.1016/j.fcl.2016.04.012   **foot.theclinics.com**
1083-7515/16/$ – see front matter © 2016 Elsevier Inc. All rights reserved.

Diabetes is the most common cause of peripheral neuropathy globally. The prevalence of diabetic Charcot neuroarthropathy (CN) varies from 0.08% to 7.5%,[4] increasing to 13% when considering high-risk patients referred to specialized centers.[4,5]

Diabetes is the leading cause of nontraumatic lower limb amputation,[6] with diabetic foot ulcers preceding more than 80% to 84% of amputations.[7,8]

The relative risk of ulcer occurrence is between 1.93 and 2.56 among diabetic patients with deformities as compared with individuals with no or few deformities.[9,10]

The "epidemic of diabetes," first described by Zimmet in 1992,[11] continues to increase. The complications of diabetes, which include diabetic foot syndrome (DFS): ulcers, infection, and destruction of the deep tissues of the foot with non-healing wounds,[12] and CN, result in an increasing "economic burden and human suffering."[13]

In 2015, the International Diabetes Federation (IDF) estimated 450 million people currently live with diabetes. The 2040 prediction is currently an estimated 642 million people[3] (**Table 1**).

Foot complications are common in people with diabetes. It is estimated that 10% of people with diabetes will have a diabetic foot ulcer at some point in their lives, with a lifetime incidence of developing an ulcer of 15% to 25%.[1]

The multidisciplinary "team approach," with patient education and surveillance at its core, has contributed significantly to the downward trend of limb-threatening complication rates.[10] However, the aim of reducing the incidence of amputations and mortality associated with this disease process[14] is impeded by the continued increase

Table 1
Estimated prevalence of diabetes

Country	2015 Prevalence	Country	2040 Prevalence
Saudi Arabia	20.0	Saudi Arabia	20.8
Qatar	20.0	Qatar	20.3
Kuwait	20.0	Kuwait	19.8
Bahrain	19.6	Bahrain	19.8
United Arab Emirates	19.3	United Arab Emirates	19.8
Malaysia	17.9	Malaysia	18.3
Egypt	16.7	Egypt	17.6
Belize	16.5	Belize	16.8
Mexico	15.8	Mexico	16.3
Oman	14.8	Oman	15.4
Brunei Darussalam	13.7	Brunei Darussalam	13.6
Caribbean	10.4–13.5	Caribbean	10.7–14.5
Turkey	12.8	Turkey	13.0
United States	10.8	United States	10.5
Singapore	10.5	Singapore	10.5
Brazil	10.4	Brazil	10.4
India	9.3	India	10.1
Russia	9.2	Russia	9.3
China	8.0	China	10.1
United Kingdom	4.7	United Kingdom	4.8

Data from International Diabetes Federation. IDF diabetes atlas. 7th edition. Brussels (Belgium): International Diabetes Federation; 2015. Available at: http://www.diabetesatlas.org.

in the "at-risk" population. Thus, the vision of the IDF of "living in a world without diabetes" is still a long way off.

Wound healing is often a protracted process, commonly punctuated by recurrence during the first 2 months after closure.[9] For the patient, this requires multiple weekly visits to hospital. This impact on work and family life is significant and can lead to increased social isolation. Unsurprisingly, patients with diabetic foot ulcers are at risk of low mood and self-esteem. Consequently, the patient may be less vigilant with regards to their diet and glycemic control, finding it difficult to take regular exercise and give up smoking. Thus, the vicious cycle of ulceration is perpetuated.

Cost

Diabetes is a significant challenge for health care systems and an obstacle to sustainable economic development due to an increased use of health services and loss of productivity.[3]

Twelve percent of global health expenditure, US$673 billion, is spent on diabetes. This amount is expected to increase to 19%, nearly US$800 billion, by 2040.[3] Most countries spend between 5% and 20% of their total health expenditure on diabetes.[3] For the National Health Service (NHS) in England and Wales, £650 million (or £1 of every £150 the NHS spends) is spent on foot ulcers or amputations each year.[1]

This large financial burden is distributed among primary and community care, outpatient costs, increased bed occupancy, and prolonged stays in hospital, with long-term support needed to overcome diabetes-related complications, such as kidney failure, blindness, and cardiac problems.

Most physicians and patients agree that prevention of lower extremity ulceration, infection, and amputation is the most desirable clinical and cost-effective strategy.[15] An effective screening program of £100 per patient per year can produce savings of 11 amputations in 1000 patients at a cost of £12,084 per amputation.[15]

When surgery is indicated, the cost of limb salvage may be slightly more expensive at $56,712 vs amputation costs of $49,251; however, the latter requires prolonged inpatient rehabilitation.[16]

Quality of Life

The established view of a favorable outcome for DFS is a stable plantigrade foot, free of ulceration and infection.[14]

Dalla Paola[17] raises the question, "Does successful correction of the acquired deformity allow patients more independence?" and further suggests that "if the answer is yes, the next questions are (1) will it lead to a longer survival? (2) will it lead to an improved quality of life?."

The negative impact on health-related quality of life for patients with DFS may be as severe as in similar patients with lower extremity amputation.[18] CN has an extremely negative impact in terms of disability, morbidity, and quality of life in diabetic patients who suffer from this condition.[19–24]

Some experts have witnessed correction of deformity in patients with CN, greatly improving quality of life, giving greater walking independence, and potentially improving longevity. Detractors suggest that surgery is not justified given the cost of care and the risks associated with its complexity.[17]

Mortality

Mortalities after diabetic foot ulceration and amputation per se prove that lower limb amputation is not a benign outcome for any patient.[25] The life expectancy of people with diabetes is shortened by up to 15 years with 75% dying secondary to macrovascular complications.[3]

Mortality in the diabetic population at 1 to 2 years following transtibial amputation is between 25% and 36%, and up to 70% at 5 years,[26,27] with diabetic patients having a 55% greater risk of death following amputation than nondiabetics.

The median survival in diabetics is 40% less than for the nondiabetic amputee at only 27.2 months following amputation.[25] The short-term mortality is primarily related to cardiac events, with rates ranging from 28.5% to 52.2%.[26,28] The increased exertion of gait required after amputation is considered to be the most likely cause.

Within the diabetic population, mortalities vary. Diabetes with no foot abnormality has the lowest mortality. Ischemic ulceration, secondary to peripheral and macrovascular disease,[29] has the highest 5-year mortality and shortest median time to death, compared with purely neuropathic and mixed neuroischemic ulcers.[30]

Interestingly, in the neuropathic group, ulceration alone has a higher mortality than when the neuropathic ulcer is associated with a CN deformity. And may be due to multiorgan failure and subsequent death. Of deaths, 14.2% to 26.1% are secondary to the adverse systemic effects of infection and subsequent sepsis (**Table 2**).[26,28,31]

The higher mortality associated with digital amputations may be due to these patients having greater comorbidities and potentially being at greater risk from general anesthetic.

Amputation

Amputation rates are 10 to 30 times higher in the diabetic population than the general population.[18,34] After a first amputation, people with diabetes are twice as likely to have a subsequent amputation as people without diabetes.[1]

Within the diabetic population, the risk of amputation is different depending on the cause of the ulcer.

Purely neuropathic ulcers have a lower 5-year risk of amputation[30] than combined neuroischemic or purely ischemic ulcers, but still have a 7% risk of amputation at 10 years.[35]

CN per se does not significantly increase the risk of amputation (<2%).[36] In fact, the risk of amputation secondary to CN is 7-fold less than in patients with diabetic foot ulcer.[36] As long as the foot remains plantigrade and the radiographic relationship between the hindfoot and forefoot remains collinear, the risk of developing an ulcer remains low. Therefore, early surgical intervention for CN in the absence of deformity or ulceration may not be advisable.[36] However, when protective footwear is no longer able to control the abnormal deforming forces,[29] a background of CN with ulceration or underlying osteomyelitis increases the risk of amputation and death significantly for the patient.[20,36–38]

Table 2				
Level of the initial amputation also significant influences mortality risk				
Level of Amputation		**30-d Mortality (%)**	**1-y Mortality (%)**	**5-y Mortality (%)**
Minor	Digit	—	6.6	26.2
	Ray	—	4.4	15.8
	Midfoot	—	10.5	21
Major	Below knee	3.6–4.2	18.2	36
	Above knee	17.5		

Data from Refs.[14,32,33]

PATHOGENESIS
Development of Ulcer

The pathogenesis of the diabetic foot ulcer is multifactorial and is the combination of altered sensation, biomechanics, hard, dry skin, and sluggish vascularity.

Peripheral neuropathy has been identified as the major contributing cause of ulcer formation in 78% of ulcers. Mechanical foot deformities come a close second at 63%, and peripheral vascular disease is present in 35%.[39,40] Individually, any one of these contributes to the formation of ulcers but may not be sufficient in isolation to cause acute ulceration.[39] The presence of 2 or more risk factors increases the risk of ulceration between 35% and 78% depending on the component risk factors, and a "clinical triad" of neuropathy, minor foot trauma, and foot deformity is present in more than 63% of patients who developed an ulcer.[39]

Neuropathy in diabetes involves the motor, sensory, and the autonomic pathways.[39] Large- and small-fiber neuropathy, proximal motor and acute mononeuropathies, and pressure palsies can exist in isolation or collectively.[24]

Sensory neuropathy causes an insensate foot with loss of protective pain, pressure, and temperature, increasing the likelihood of repetitive trauma.[20]

Brand[41] observed that the first stage of ulcer formation is an inflammatory state causing an increase in local skin temperature. The normal vasodilator response to the painful stimuli of injury or inflammation is impaired in diabetic neuropathy by impeding the C-receptor-dependent nerve axon reflex.[42]

Uncontrolled inflammation via a neurally mediated vascular reflex leads to increased peripheral blood flow and active bone resorption in the foot.[20] The continual production of proinflammatory cytokines and osteoclasts results in osteolysis. The osteoclasts have been shown to be more aggressive due to increased resorptive ability.[43] When combined with repeated microtrauma, ulceration is the outcome.

Autonomic dysfunction causes vasodilation and decreased sweating, resulting in dry warm feet. Hard dry skin, prone to cracking, facilitates infection. Bergtholdt and Brand[44,45] postulated that if this area before breakdown is effectively managed, permanent injury may be avoided.[46]

Motor nerve involvement causes an abnormal gait due to motor weakness and decreased muscle mass. Abnormal pressure on the foot causes a hypertrophic reactive response and callus formation. Removal of callus reduces the dynamic plantar pressures in the forefoot by 30%.[29]

The changes in biomechanics of the foot are further potentiated due to glycation of collagen in the tissues,[47–49] causing cheiroarthropathy (stiff joints) due to retraction of the intrinsic muscle of the foot, with the subsequent development of hammer and claw toes. Hammer and claw toes can result in rubbing on the plantar tip of the toe with thickening of the toenail, causing additional pressure areas. The dorsal aspect of the proximal interphalangeal joint rubbing against ill-fitting shoes results in wound breakdown. A similar mechanism is responsible for the contracture of the Achilles tendon, causing an increased pressure area on any of the metatarsal heads, resulting in skin breakdown and subsequent development of an ulcer.

In CN, the bony deformity is due to a combination of motor neuropathy[50] and reduction in calcitonin gene-related peptide released from nerve terminals, which is responsible for the maintenance of the normal integrity of the joint capsule,[51] and, indirectly, osteolysis. The combination results in the progressive fracture and dislocation that characterize its presentation.[52]

Ischemic ulceration is caused by a combination of alteration in blood vessel structure and function. Both microvascular and the macrovascular disease of peripheral arterial disease are present in the diabetic patient.

The microcirculatory problems of the foot may be more functional in that some patients with severe disease have been shown to have normal capillaries on skin or skeletal muscle biopsy.[39]

Impaired Healing

The same factors that initially cause the ulcer are also responsible for the inability of the ulcer to heal. Diabetes affects all systems, and patients may have associated nephropathies, retinopathies, heart disease, renal failure, which contribute to the outcome of the healing ulcer. High glucose levels in tissues, malnutrition, and immunodeficiency increase the risk of infection.[53–55]

DIAGNOSIS
Diabetic Foot Ulcer

According to the 2015 National Institute for Health and Care Excellence guidelines,[1] the diagnosis of a diabetic ulcer should include a standardized system of assessment, for example, the SINBAD (Site, Ischemia, Neuropathy, Bacterial infection, Area, and Depth) or the University of Texas classification system to document the size, depth and position, and severity of the foot ulcer.

Charcot Neuroarthropathy

The diagnosis of CN requires a high index of suspicion and is essentially one of exclusion until proven otherwise. The challenge in the diabetic patient who presents with a markedly swollen, erythematous foot, with a history of neuropathy, is being able to differentiate osteomyelitis from CN. Clinically, a temperature difference greater than 2°, with minimal pain and bounding pulses in a neuropathic foot, make CN more likely.

INVESTIGATIONS

Initially there are 2 questions that need to be asked when first presented with a diabetic foot ulcer, because the subsequent management may be different:

1. What type of ulcer is this: ischemic, neuropathic, or mixed?
2. Is this CN until proved otherwise, or osteomyelitis (**Table 3**)?

Table 3 Assessment of arterial blood supply	
Assessment	**Relevance**
Pedal pulses	Good volume and pressure pedal pulses precludes a diagnosis of arterial disease
Ankle-brachial index (ABI) (normal index of 0.9–1.3)	May be falsely elevated or normal, even in the presence of arterial disease due to noncompressible vessels secondary to atherosclerotic calcification
Toe pressures	Better test of vascularity than ABIs
Doppler ultrasound	Dampened waves on in the presence of normal ABI suggest calcified vessels and should be further investigated
MR angiography	Most accurate in diagnosing arterial disease as blood flow at velocities as low as 2 cm/s can be measured[23]

Osteomyelitis Versus Charcot Neuroarthropathy

Osteomyelitis continues to be a confounding factor in the diagnosis of acute CN. No single investigation is the gold standard. The development of new techniques, such as hybrid PET, has shown some promise in this regard[60] (**Table 4**).

Table 4
Assessment of osteomyelitis versus Charcot neuroarthropathy

Assessment	Relevance	
Clinical assessment	Osteomyelitis affects a single bone in the forefoot or hindfoot, whereas CN affects many bones, commonly in the midfoot[56]	
Plain radiograph	Signs of osteomyelitis may be lacking in the first few weeks, because it takes 30%–50% bone loss before they become evident on radiographs[17]	
MRI	Radiograph inconclusive and ulceration with high likelihood of deep infection No metalwork present MRI, with a sensitivity of 90%–100% and specificity of 80%–100%,[17] can detect subtle early changes differentiating between CN and osteomyelitis	
	Osteomyelitis	**CN**
	Low signal intensity only on T_1-weighted and high signal intensity on T_2-weighted images. The edema is on one side of the joint and not confined to the juxta-articular area[57]	Low signal intensity in subchondral bone on both T1- and T2-weighted images, which correlates with sclerosis on radiographs. The edema is localized to the juxta-articular region[57]
Triple-phase bone scan, combined with white-labeled scan	Useful when MRI is inconclusive or metalwork present[17,20]	
Bone mineral density (BMD)		Pathologic pattern of CN shows joint dislocation is more prevalent in those with normal BMD vs fracture in those with diminished BMD[58]
Bone biopsy	Gold standard for diagnosis of osteomyelitis Lesions that extend more than 2 cm^2 Positive "probe-to-bone" test Erythrocyte sedimentation rate of more than 70 mm/h has a positive predictive value of 89%[42,59] Deep soft tissue and bone should be sent for analysis, because soft tissue pathogens may not always reflect the organism involved in the underlying osteomyelitis[81]	

Radiographic Classification of Charcot Neuroarthropathy

The 5 D's of joint distension, dislocation, debris, disorganization, and increased density[61] are the essence of the original description of the 3 phases by Eichenholtz[62] (**Table 5**).

Many investigators have attempted to create a definitive anatomic classification (**Tables 6** and **7**).

With the midfoot being the most common site for Charcot, both Easley and Schon have further divided the midtarsus deformities[63,65] (**Tables 8** and **9**).

Foot ulceration is more likely in sagittal plane deformities than transverse plane deformities. Lateral column involvement (assessed by cuboid height, decreased calcaneal pitch, and decreased lateral calcaneal fifth metatarsal angle) is associated with a worse prognosis than medial column involvement (assessed by lateral talar-first metatarsal angle and medial column height)[66] (**Table 10**).

MANAGEMENT
Conservative Treatment

Central to this team are the diabetic podiatrist and orthotist, who have developed successful pathways to monitor the risk of, and conservative management of, ulceration (**Box 1**).

Microbiological Tests and Antimicrobial Agents

During debridement, deep tissue culture should be taken.[67,68,70] If infection is confirmed, 4 to 6 weeks of parenteral antibiotics, which should cover for *Staphylococcus* due to its high prevalence, should be administered in conjunction with surgical debridement for the eradication of osteomyelitis.[44]

Off-Loading the Neuropathic Ulcer

Brand[41] famously said, "Pain is God's greatest gift to mankind." The pioneer of total contact casting, Brand confirmed the relationship between repetitive pressure and ulceration in the insensitive limb.

If a plantigrade foot can be achieved and maintained, greater than 50% of neuropathic ulcers can be treated nonsurgically.[71] Offloading ranges from strict bed rest

Table 5
Eichenholtz original radiographic classification with Shibata modification
Eichenholtz Stage 1–4 **Original Staging System Based on Clinical and Radiograph Findings** **Shibata Stage 0** **An Earlier, Fourth Stage**
Stage 0 Absence of injury or osteoarticular disorders[64]
Stage 1 Acute phase. Inflammation, erythema, swelling, and a temperature difference present clinically Fracture or dislocation may be subtle initially but later the calcaneal inclination angle is reduced and the talo-first metatarsal angle is broken with calcification of the medial arteries evident[50]
Stage 2 Coalescence or subacute phase; reduction in temperature, swelling, and inflammation A reparative process is seen on radiograph
Stage 3 Consolidation or chronic phase Inflammation has completely resolved and the fractures consolidated[62]

Table 6
Sanders and Frykberg anatomic classification

Five Locations with Associated Frequency of Onset	
Type I	Forefoot (15%)
Type II	TMT joint (40%)
Type III	Naviculocuneiform/talonavicular/calcaneocuboid joints (30%)
Type VI	Ankle and/or subtalar joint (10%)
Type V	Calcaneus (5%)

Data from Sanders LJ, Frykberg RG. Diabetic neuropathic osteoarthropathy: the Charcot foot. In: Frykberg RG, editor. The high risk foot in diabetes mellitus. New York: Churchill Livingstone; 1991. p. 297–338.

to specialized footwear. It must be used consistently and demands good patient compliance. The best off-loading device is a non-removable, total contact cast (TCC).[72,73] However, it is technically demanding, and if wrongly applied, can prolong ulceration. Healing in the early phase (6–8 weeks) is with skin that it is still fragile. Patients can gradually move to custom footwear with full-length shoe total contact insert to provide pressure reduction.[74–77]

Risk of Recurrence

The risk of recurrence after healing with conservative treatment ranges from 12% to 33%,[78] with the risk of reulceration at 5 years as high as 70% in patients with diabetic foot ulcer.[79,80] In acute Charcot arthropathy, 7% to 15% reulceration rates have been quoted.[67,68]

Avoid Smoking and Tobacco

Smoking is a risk factor because of its effects of vessel constriction (short term) and the enhanced development of atherosclerosis (long term).[39] Wound healing is impaired by reduced O_2 delivery to the wound site, and the toxic effect of nicotine, carbon monoxide, and hydrogen cyanide on platelets inhibits normal cellular metabolism.[39,81,84]

When the patient first presents, if there is no temperature or if the foot is hot and swollen, MRI is performed to differentiate between osteomyelitis and CN (**Table 11**).

Table 7
Brodsky anatomic classification

Addresses the Question of Stability, but Does Not Differentiate the Various Mid-tarsal Patterns or Severity	
Type 1	Midfoot deformity (70%); most stable; rocker-bottom foot with bony prominences and plantar ulceration
Type 2	Hindfoot/subtalar/talonavicular/calcaneocuboid joints (20%)
Type 3a	Ankle associated with disintegration of the talus (5%); most unstable type; associated varus or valgus; may cause malleolar ulceration
Type 3b	Pathologic fracture of the calcaneus (5%)

Breakdown of soft tissues from bony prominences occurred most commonly in the type I pattern and these ulcers were located on the plantar surface of the foot.[99]
Data from Brodsky JW. The diabetic foot. In: Mann RA, Coughlin MJ, editors. Surgery of the foot and ankle. 6th edition. St Louis (MO): Mosby-YearBook Inc; 1993. p. 877–958.

Table 8	
Schon midfoot classification	
Schon	
Type I	TMT joints often associated with forefoot abduction
Type II	Naviculocuneiform joints medially; fourth and fifth metatarsocuboid joints laterally; plantar prominence begins laterally and progresses medially
Type III	Collapse or fragmentation of the navicular; supination and adduction of the foot
Type IV	Transverse tarsal joints; plantar prominence under the calcaneocuboid joint or talonavicular joint
Schon also assigned an alpha stage (no additional features) and beta stage, where one of the following 4 criteria are met:	
Beta 1	Dislocation is present
Beta 2	Lateral talar-first metatarsal angle is 30°
Beta 3	Lateral calcaneal-fifth metatarsal angle 0°
Beta 4	Anteroposterior talar-first metatarsal angle is 35°

Data from Schon LC, Easley ME, Cohen I, et al. The acquired midtarsus deformity classification system-interobserver reliability and intraobserver reproducibility. Foot Ankle Int 2002;23(1):30–6; and Schon LC, Easley ME, Weinfeld SB. Charcot neuroarthropathy of the foot and ankle. Clin Orthop 1998(349):116–31.

SURGERY

Surgery for this group of patients is clinically challenging and one of the most controversial issues facing orthopedic foot and ankle surgeons. Patients often have multiple medical comorbidities and may be obese, making use of cumbersome orthoses difficult.[71,73] Published algorithms are based almost entirely on level 4 or 5 evidence.[85] Questions remain around the timing of surgery, the best surgical approach and construct, the adjuncts to surgery, and the postoperative rehabilitation.

The aim of surgery is to enable the patient to maintain walking independence using commercially available depth-inlay shoes and custom accommodative orthoses.[85–87] The threshold for achieving a successful outcome becomes far more difficult when the desired endpoint is use of commercially available, non-custom-fabricated, depth-inlay therapeutic footwear and custom orthotic insoles.[73]

Table 9	
Easley midfoot classification	
Easley	
Distinct Clinical and Biomechanical Features to Distinguish Between Metatarsocuneiform, Cuneiform-Navicular Perinavicular, and Transverse Tarsal (Chopart) Sites of Collapse. Four Angles are Measured.	
Two lateral	Talar-first metatarsal reflecting the medial arch collapse
	Calcaneo-fifth metatarsal reflecting the lateral arch collapse
Two anteroposterior	Talar-first metatarsal correlating with the degree of abduction
	Talonavicular coverage signifying the severity of transverse tarsal collapse

It was also noted that hindfoot involvement of the Chopart joints contributes to both the rockerbottom deformity and the varus/valgus deformities.

Data from Schon LC, Easley ME, Cohen I, et al. The acquired midtarsus deformity classification system-interobserver reliability and intraobserver reproducibility. Foot Ankle Int 2002;23(1):30–6.

Table 10
Selia anatomic and management classification
Five Stages of Charcot Deformities, Based on Radiographs and Bone Scan, with a Recommended Treatment Plan for Each Stage
Stage 0   Edema, increase temperature, pain Radiographs are negative Technetium 99 bone scan is markedly positive Limited weight-bearing and close observation are required
Stage 1   Periarticular cysts, erosions, localized osteopenia, and sometimes diastases are seen on radiographs Total contact casting is followed by a University of California Biomechanics Lab orthosis, to maintain the arch while allowing limited weight-bearing
Stage 2   Marked joint subluxations between the second cuneiform and the base of the second metatarsal and spreading laterally Partial weight-bearing in TCC is followed by a Charcot restraint orthotic walker (CROW) Surgery may be needed at this stage, while the joints are still reducible. Arthrodesis with rigid fixation is recommended
Stage 3   Joint dislocation and arch collapse Casting for the acute phase, then with a patellar-tendon–bearing ankle-foot orthosis or CROW If ulcers are present, treat with weekly local debridement, antibiotics, and total contact casting. Occasionally decompressive ostectomy is required
Stage 4   Healed and stable No temperature gradient between the 2 feet Trabeculation across joint spaces indicative of mature fusion Bony prominences causing the nonhealing ulcers may need surgical removal[69]

Data from Sella EJ, Barrette C. Staging of Charcot neuroarthropathy along the medial column of the foot in the diabetic patient. J Foot Ankle Surg 1999;38(1):34–40.

Depending on the clinical situation, this can be achieved surgically in many ways[17] (**Table 12**).

A group of orthopedic foot and ankle surgeons has emerged that believes surgical reconstruction in CN should not be limited to a salvage procedure but an alternative to amputation.[88,89] Selected patients with nonplantigrade feet, instability, and manifest

Box 1
UK National Institute for Health and Care Excellence guidelines 2015
• Good diabetic control and pressure-redistribution to minimize risk of pressure ulcers developing
• Once a diabetic foot ulcer has developed, offloading with non-removable casting should be used with dressings to control foot infection
• Wound debridement in hospital should only be done by health care professionals from the multidisciplinary foot care service
• For diabetic patients with peripheral neuropathy, high index of suspicion, in those who experience pain or edema without a history of trauma. These patients should be promptly offloaded until the diagnosis is confirmed[14]
From NICE–Diabetic foot problems: preventions and management. NICE Guideline. 2015.

Table 11	
Management of diabetic foot ulcer	

Systemically well	Systemically unwell
Outpatient diabetic foot clinic	Admit as inpatient under Medicine/Vascular

Microbiology

Swab ulcer/tissue sample/bone biopsy are taken and antibiotics started only once cultures are grown

Off-loading

Focal differences of >4° detected, off-loaded the foot in a TTC until the temperature returns to normal (usually 2–4 d, around 4 wk but may be longer)[82]
Initial offloading management is with TCC. This is removed and checked at day 3
Weekly cast changes until edema has resolved the temperature within 2°.[83]
Edema reduction most marked in the first few weeks during which the patient should be non-weight-bearing.[83]

Radiograph

Radiographs are taken at weekly intervals to assess for the development of any deformity

Normal radiograph	Calcification of vessels on radiograph	
	Any suggestion of an ischemic component to the ulcer vascular investigations	
Abnormal sensation	Abnormal sensation	Normal sensation
Good pulses	Poor/absent pulses	Poor/absent pulses

Ulcer type

Neuropathic	Neuroischemic	Ischemic
	Vascular assessment	
	Doppler, MR angiogram	
	Interventional angioplasty	
	Vascular surgery	
	Angioplasty/bypass	

Osteomyelitis/CN

No metalwork	Metalwork
MRI	White-labeled nuclear medicine scan

Off-load with TTC

Antibiotics (up to 6 wk) if infection present

Surgical correction of deformity
NEMISIS

Postoperatively

Oral antibiotics for 1–2 wk postoperatively

Below knee cast with Bholer walker for 3 mo

± US bone stimulator

Change to moonboot with TTC insole

Fitted for custom shoes with TTC insole

or impending ulcers may benefit from early surgical reconstruction with long-lasting functional improvement and without recurrence of instability or ulceration.[90]

Timing of Surgery

In the acute stage of CN, the foot is warm. A temperature difference between the feet of 2°C is considered significant. This temperature can be measured using an infrared thermometer.[7,8] Furthermore, a temperature difference of less than 2°C between the limbs is used as a determinant of the end of the acute phase.[6,34,35,91]

Table 12 Surgical options	
Debridement	The surgical removal of infected or necrotic tissue from below and/or around a wound with underlying osteomyelitis
Conservative surgery	The removal of infected bone and surrounding soft tissues
Minor amputations	Amputation of a portion of the foot below the ankle joint
Major amputations	Amputation proximal to the ankle joint

Data from Dalla Paola L. Confronting a dramatic situation: the Charcot foot complicated by osteomyelitis. Int J Low Extrem Wounds 2014;13(4):247–62.

Benefits from early surgical intervention in high-risk patients are potentially shorter in duration for treatment with an improved quality of life, with an overall reduction in cost.[26] However, although surgical intervention during the acute phase of CN is encouraging, the evidence comparing early versus late surgery is currently inconclusive.[85]

Because of an increased risk of infection,[92] some advocate delaying surgery until the ulcer has definitely healed,[89,93,94] or using external fixators.[86] However, it has been shown that even in the presence of an open wound, one-stage corrective arthrodesis can heal these ulcers, with no major increase in the risk for complications.[90] Therefore, there is probably little to be gained from delaying surgery, unless for optimizing the patient's comorbidities.

SURGICAL OPTIONS
Correction of Equinus

Equinus deformity secondary to a contracted tendo-Achilles (TA) creates a bending moment, which may be responsible for the location of the acquired deformity at the midfoot level, in more than 85% of patients.[20,73]

TA tendon lengthening or gastrocnemius muscle recession reduces forefoot pressure, establishing muscle balance between the ankle flexor and extensor muscles, improving the alignment of the ankle and hindfoot to the midfoot and forefoot.[14,73,85] Removal of the equinus deforming force combined with TCC can significantly reduce the incidence of ulcer recurrence, when compared with TCC alone (15% vs 59% at 7 months).[50,95–98]

Flexor tenotomies have also been suggested to decrease metatarsal head ulcers in patients with claw toes.[98]

Exostectomy

In Charcot arthropathy, joint subluxation and dislocation cause bony prominences, which are not true exostoses.[60] Provided the midfoot is stable, particularly in patients without ulceration, exostectomy is good at relieving mechanical pressures that are unable to be accommodated by orthotics.[14,20,60,73,85,99]

Arthrodesis

The most common location requiring surgical intervention for CN patients is the midfoot (59%).[85]

Surgical correction of deformity is advised when patients have a nonplantigrade foot or developed such a deformity during treatment.[71]

Despite a high rate of incomplete union, arthrodesis is a good option for patients who fail nonoperative treatment and present with instability pain or recurrent ulceration.[14,85]

Fixation

Inconclusive data exist recommending one form of fixation over another, that is, internal versus external, or plating over intramedullary beaming.[14,85] Although there is a slight trend to a stiffer construct with plantar plating, there is no statistical biomechanical difference between tarsometatarsal (TMT) joint fusion with plantar plating versus intramedullary screw fixation.[100]

External fixators have the advantages of permitting the monitoring of soft tissue healing and avoidance of more invasive surgery in patients with infection.[101–103] However, the complication of pin tract infection has prompted some to recommend a staged minimally invasive technique, with initial gradual distraction using an external fixator followed by arthrodesis with percutaneous internal fixation.[104]

The "superconstructs" described by Sammarco[105] combines plantar locking plating and axial screw fixation to provide further stability.

Thus, implant choice for arthrodesis remains at the surgeon's discretion, because none has been proven superior to the others.[60]

Beaming

In 1997, Grant and colleagues[106,107] presented the concept of beaming to provide lateral and medial column stability, using large intramedullary (6.5–8.0 mm) cannulated screws, combined with arthrodesis of the subtalar joint.

By extending the arthrodesis beyond the affected zone to include nonaffected joints, these superconstructs reduce the deformity while protecting the soft tissues by shortening the extremity.[78]

Theoretically, beaming provides anatomic realignment of the columns and the transverse arch of the foot.

The medial column runs through the medullary canal of the first metatarsal, medial cuneiform, and navicular, into the body of the talus. The lateral column beam runs from the space between the bases of the third and fourth metatarsals, then across the calcaneocuboid joint, and into the body of the calcaneus.[106]

Fusion of the subtalar joint may add further stability by limiting transverse and frontal plane torsion.[106]

These "reinforcement rods" confer elastic and tensile strength to the diseased bone and ligamentous structures found in the diabetic neuropathic foot. The beam accepts the axial forces of compression and tension, sharing the load with the bones, ligaments, and joints of the foot decreasing the bending forces on the bone.[106]

By beaming both the medial and the lateral columns, control of the transverse arch is achieved, providing maximal stability to the hindfoot and Lisfranc Charcot joints.[108–110]

One-Stage Approach

A plantigrade, stable foot, which remains ulcer free, can be achieved as a one-stage procedure.[90] Irrespective of whether it is a bony or fibrous union that is achieved, patients accomplished full weight-bearing within a mean of 3.5 months after surgery.[90,111]

Complications

With a one-stage procedure, the rate of hardware failure with nonunion[112–115] can be high (0%–30%). However, this does not necessarily correlate with progression of deformity or subsequent amputation. Stable fibrous nonunion in good position does not necessarily require surgery.[90] The deep infection rate after primary arthrodesis is lower than that for secondary arthrodesis, where the infection rate ranges from 0% to more than 30%.[90]

Neuropathic Minimally Invasive Surgeries

The decision of when to operate is the most challenging aspect (**Table 13**). In the author's hospital, this is done as part of the multidisciplinary diabetic foot and ankle team, which is headed by a consultant diabetologist, with diabetic podiatrist and orthotist and input from consultant interventional radiologist, consultant microbiologist, consultant vascular surgeon, and consultant orthopedic foot and ankle surgeon. Patients who have recurrence of ulcer, deformity that is at risk of ulceration, or progression of joint destruction on serial radiographs are considered for neuropathic minimally invasive surgeries (NEMISIS) surgical stabilization (**Box 2**).

Once listed for surgery, the diabetologist works closely with the anesthetist to ensure that the patient is optimized medically for surgery (**Table 14**).

FOREFOOT SURGERY
Preoperative Planning

Preoperative radiographs and MRI scans are performed to assess for any evidence of osteomyelitis or malalignment of the forefoot.

Admission and Anesthesia

The patient is admitted as a day case. Surgery is performed under general anesthesia with popliteal block and intravenous antibiotics after bone and soft tissue biopsies (usually flucloxacillin and gentamicin, depending on previous sensitivities, allergies, and renal function).

Surgical Setup

- The patient is placed on the operating table with the feet off the end of the bed, to allow for easy access of the mini-C arm.
- The operating table should be positioned in the theater with the *feet* centered under the operating lights, to ensure that there is sufficient space for the mini-C arm and equipment.
- The mini-C arm is used for intraoperative fluoroscopy, which should come in from the end of the bed, for maximum maneuverability.
- Calf tourniquet (if pulses present).

Step 1
Step 1 includes assessment of TA tightness. If the foot is not plantigrade due to tightness within the TA, a percutaneous TA lengthening is performed.

Step 2
Step 2 involves assessment of the lesser toes (**Table 15**). Lesser toes are assessed for deformity, especially fixed deformities, that have increased risk of ulceration.

Step 3
Step 3 involves debridement of the fifth metatarsal osteomyelitis (**Fig. 1**). Osteooyelitis requires removal of all infected and dead bone with the burr, followed by extensive irrigation.

MIDFOOT CORRECTION
Preoperative Planning

Computed tomography, with 3-dimensional reconstructions, is useful to determine the planes for the osteotomies. MRI is used to determine if any osteomyelitis is present.

Table 13
Neuropathic minimally invasive surgeries surgical options

Greater Toe Surgery

No Achilles Contracture	Achilles Contracture
Conservative	Percutaneous TA lengthening/medial gastrocnemius recession
No osteomyelitis	Osteomyelitis / Not responding to antibiotics
Conservative	Minimally invasive surgery (MIS) debridement & antibiotics for 1–6 wk
Joint preserved no deformity	Joint preserved Deformity — Joint destroyed Deformity
Conservative	Flexor or extensor tenotomies / P1 osteotomies / DMMO — MIS IPJ fusion or MIS MTP joint fusion / Dorsiflexion osteotomies/ 1st TMT joint arthrodesis

Lesser Toe Surgery

No Achilles Contracture	Achilles Contracture
Conservative	Percutaneous TA lengthening/medial gastrocnemius recession
No osteomyelitis	Osteomyelitis / Not responding to antibiotics
Conservative	MIS debridement & antibiotics for 1–6 wk debridement
Joint preserved No deformity	Joint preserved Deformity — Joint destroyed Deformity
Conservative	Flexor or extensor tenotomies / P1, P2 osteotomies / DMMO — DMMO / Debridement of IPJ / Debridement of metatarsal head

Midfoot Surgery

No Achilles Contracture	Achilles Contracture
Conservative	Percutaneous TA lengthening/medial gastrocnemius recession
No osteomyelitis	Osteomyelitis / Not responding to antibiotics
Conservative	MIS debridement & antibiotics for 1–6 wk
Joint preserved no deformity	Joint destroyed or deformity / MIS midfoot joint arthrodesis / With beaming
Conservative	

Hindfoot Surgery

No Achilles Contracture	Achilles Contracture
Conservative	Percutaneous TA lengthening/medial gastrocnemius recession
No osteomyelitis	Osteomyelitis / Not responding to antibiotics
Conservative	MIS debridement & antibiotics for 1–6 wk
Joint preserved, no deformity	Joint destroyed or deformity / MIS subtalar arthrodesis / MIS TTC nail
Conservative	

Box 2
Neuropathic Minimally Invasive Surgeries principles

- Percutaneous incisions minimize damage to the soft tissues
- Percutaneous surgery is performed away from the blood vessels, thus reducing the risk of nonhealing wounds, tissue necrosis, and major amputation
- The traditional approach to ulcers that have exposed bone, tendons, and the area of the ulcer that has not decreased by more than 10% after conservative management for 2 months is plastic surgery with skin graft, and regional or free flaps.[116,117] Removal of abnormal bone relieves the tension on the soft tissues of the foot; thus, complications of wound breakdown and skin necrosis are minimized and plastic surgery may be avoided
- Stabilization of the joints with percutaneous beaming provides maintenance of correction, stability
- Restoration of the foot to as near normal biomechanical alignment as possible

Preoperative Prophylaxis

Five days of Nacetpin nasal cream and Hibiscrub is prescribed to reduce the risk of postoperative infection from *Staphylococcus.*

Admission and Anesthesia

The patient is admitted as an inpatient, and surgery is performed under general anesthesia with popliteal block and intravenous antibiotics after bone biopsies (usually flucloxacillin and gentamicin, depending on previous sensitivities, allergies, and renal function).

Surgical Setup

Surgical setup is as for forefoot surgery.

Step 1

Step 1 includes an assessment of TA tightness. If the foot is not plantigrade due to tightness within the TA, a percutaneous TA lengthening is performed.

Step 2

Two 2-mm K-wires are placed from medial to lateral to act as a guide for plantar-medial closing wedge osteotomy (**Fig. 2**).

Table 14
Assessment of the medial column

Is the great toe plantar flexed, and if so, is it fixed or flexible?	Consider dorsiflexion osteotomy of the metatarsal head or 1st TMT joint arthrodesis to reposition the metatarsal shaft
Is there pressure under the 1st metatarsal head associated with osteomyelitis?	Consider the above ± debridement of the head if any necrotic bone present
Is there hyperextension of the 1st MTP joint, and if so, is it flexible and fully correctable?	Consider z-lengthening of the extensor hallucis longus tendon, ± capsule release
Is there any evidence of joint destruction from degenerative change or significant deformity?	Consider minimally invasive 1st MTP arthrodesis, by debridement of the joint with burr and wedges, and holding with crossed 4-mm headless compression cannulated screws

Table 15
Assessment of the lesser toes

Is there any evidence of mallet/hammer or claw toe, and if so, is there any associated ulceration?	Consider flexor tenotomy, extensor tenotomy, P1 ± P2 osteotomies, or debridement of the joint with burr
Is there any prominence or ulceration of the 2nd to 5th metatarsal heads, and if so, is there any associated ulceration or evidence of osteomyelitis?	Consider DMMO to allow metatarsal head to reposition itself when weight-bearing If osteomyelitis consider debridement of metatarsal head

Step 3

Step 3 includes a dorsal longitudinal incision with Beaver blade, midway between the 2 K-wires. A 2 × 20-mm Shannon burr is used to make an osteotomy cut along the most distal K-wire, from medial to lateral. The cut often needs to be done in 2 stages, because the burr may not reach the plantar aspect of the foot on the first pass (**Fig. 3**).

The surgeon "feels" the bone to be removed under the skin Once the distal osteotomy is made, a similar cut is made along the course of the proximal wire. It is imperative that the full depth of the bone to be removed is cut and also that the osteotomy reaches right across to the lateral aspect of the foot.

Step 4

A 3.1-mm, then 4.1-mm, wedge burr is taken to convert the bone into a bone paste.

When the osteotomies have been made correctly, with sufficient removal of bone, the forefoot should now be fully mobile and able to be positioned in the correct alignment, restoring Meary angle (**Fig. 4**A–C).

If there has ever been a history of an infected ulcer, then all the bone paste should be removed and a culture sent to microbiology. If there has never been any infection, the bone paste can remain and act as bone graft. Additional bone graft can be taken from the calcaneum. Antibiotic bone graft substitute may also be added to fill the void left by the resection of the bony deformity (**Fig. 4**D).

Bone biopsies should be sent to the laboratory for histopathologic and microbiological assessment.[17]

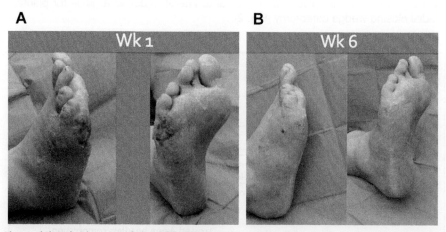

A Wk 1   **B** Wk 6

Fig. 1. (*A*) Debridement of the fifth metatarsal osteomyelitis, week 1 postoperatively. (*B*) Debridement of the fifth metatarsal osteomyelitis, week 6 postoperatively.

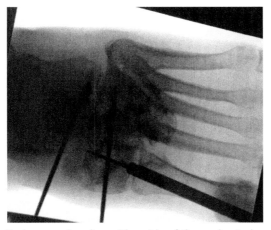

Fig. 2. Two 2-mm K-wires are placed on either side of the wedge to be resected.

Step 5

Step 5 includes 7-mm fully threaded, cannulated beams placed into the first metatarsal to talus.

There are 2 approaches.

The guidewire can either be placed retrograde through the base of the deformity, exiting at the posterior aspect of the ankle, drilled, and then the guidewire is reversed

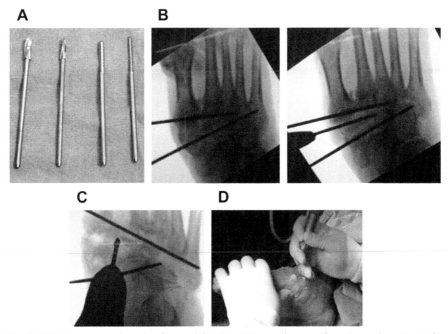

Fig. 3. (A) Shannon and wedge burrs. (B) A 2 × 20-mm Shannon burr is used to "cut" the wedge of bone. (C) 3.1-mm and 4-mm wedge burrs are then used to "mill" the bone into a paste. (D) The surgeon "feels" the bone to be removed under the skin.

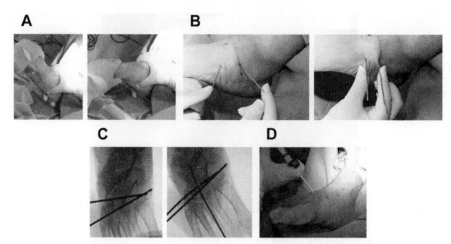

Fig. 4. (*A*) Once osteotomy is made, the distal forefoot should be fully mobile to allow it to be repositioned correctly in relation to the remaining midfoot and hindfoot. (*B*) "Joystick" K-wires to hold closing wedge osteotomy. (*C*) Before and after the "wedge" of bone has been removed. K-wires act as "joystick" for closing wedge and guidewire for screw can then be placed percutaneously. (*D*) Bone graft substitute injected into void left from removed bone "paste."

and placed antegrade from the talus to the first metatarsal. This approach avoids violating the first metatarsophalangeal joint (MTPJ; **Fig. 5**A, B). Otherwise, the guide-wire can be placed through the first metatarsal head in a similar manner to the second and third metatarsals, aiming for the talus and calcaneus. Either technique stabilizes the medial column of the foot, recreating the arch (**Fig. 5**C).

The reaming of intramedullary fixation may has a biological effect on bone healing by increasing extraosseous circulation and therefore potentially reducing the chance of nonunion.[118–121]

Step 6
Step 6 includes stabilization with 5-mm or 6.5-mm solid fusion bolts (**Fig. 6**).

Step 7
Step 7 includes reinforcing the medial column with a percutaneously placed plate if deemed necessary (**Fig. 7**).

HEEL ULCERS
Preoperative Planning

MRI is used to determine if any osteomyelitis is present.

Preoperative Prophylaxis

Five days of Nacetpin nasal cream and Hibiscrub is prescribed to reduce the risk of postoperative infection from *Staphylococcus*.

Admission and Anesthesia

The patient is admitted as a day case and surgery is performed under general anesthesia with popliteal block, and intravenous antibiotics are given after bone biopsies (usually flucloxacillin and gentamicin, depending on previous sensitivities, allergies and renal function).

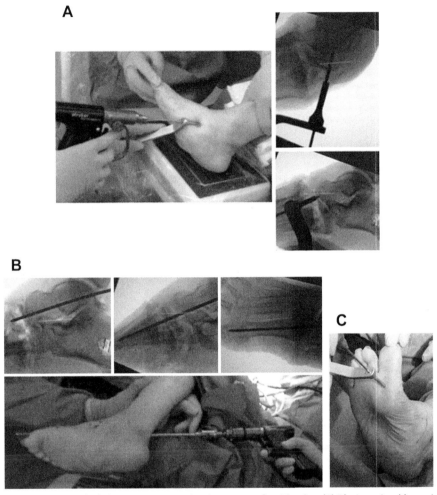

Fig. 5. (*A*) Through deformity, retrograde placement of guidewire. (*B*) The proximal bone is drilled, and the guidewire is then reversed, passed retrograde to the posterior skin, and a stab incision is made in the skin to allow retrieval of the guidewire, which is then passed antegrade into the metatarsal. (*C*) Alternatively, the guidewire can be passed retrograde through the metatarsal head to the talus.

Surgical Setup

The surgical setup is as for forefoot surgery.

Step 1
Step 1 includes assessment of the TA tightness. If the foot is not plantigrade due to tightness within the TA, a percutaneous TA lengthening is performed.

Step 2
Using a 2 × 2 Shannon and the 3.1- and 4.1-mm wedge burr, any prominent bone is removed, so that there is no mechanical pressure on the overlying skin. Versajet can be useful to remove any dead or necrotic tissue. A PICO vacuum dressing is applied after copious irrigation, and a backslab is applied.

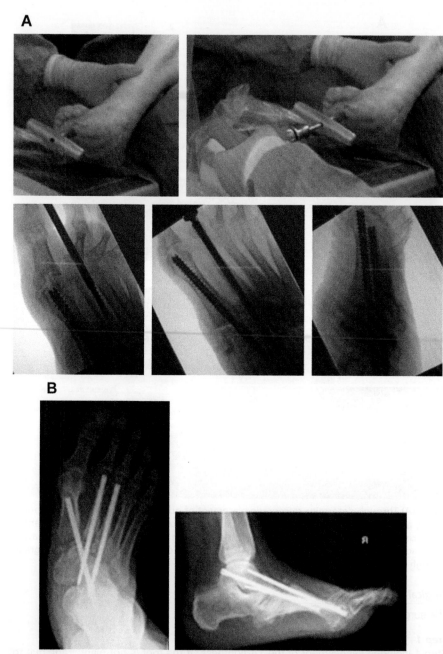

Fig. 6. (*A*) The middle column is stabilized with 5-mm or 6.5-mm solid fusion bolts. (*B*) Postoperative radiographs of stabilization of the medial and middle columns with beams and bolts.

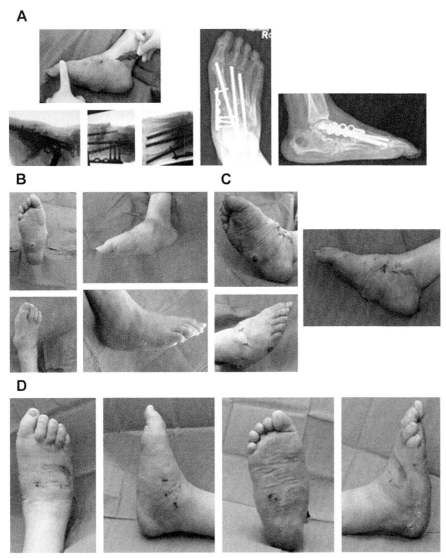

Fig. 7. (A) The medial column can be reinforced with a percutaneously placed plate if deemed necessary. (B) Preoperative correction. (C) Immediate postoperative correction. (D) Week 2 postoperative correction.

HINDFOOT CORRECTION

Preoperative planning, preoperative prophylaxis, admission, and anesthesia are all the same as for midfoot correction.

Step 1

Step 1 is to assess for TA tightness. If the foot is not plantigrade due to tightness within the TA, a percutaneous TA lengthening is performed.

Step 2

The subtalar joint is prepared via a percutaneous incision made in the midpoint of the standard incision for open subtalar fusion. The ankle joint is prepared using a percutaneous incision over the medial talar dome. Both joints are prepared using 3.1- and 4.1-mm wedge burrs. Deformity within the ankle mortice can be corrected using the wedge burr (**Fig. 8**).

Step 3

A hindfoot fusion is then placed percutaneously through the heel according as to the operating technique manual of the selected implant. Additional bone graft can be taken from the calcaneum. Antibiotic bone graft substitute may also be added to fill the void left by the resection of the bony deformity before any final compression of the hindfoot fusion nail (**Fig. 9**).

POSTOPERATIVELY

Forefoot surgery is allowed to partially weight-bear in a heel weight-bearing shoe. Midfoot and hindfoot surgery is placed into a below-knee backslab that extends beyond the toes. The patients are then seen for a wound check at 3 and 7 days. They are then placed into a full plaster cast, extending beyond the toes, with an axial off-loader (**Fig. 10**). The foot can become swollen in the early stages, with erythematous changes similar to a reactivation of CN. Burred bone and/or bone graft substitute can leak out of the incision, and thus, the patient should remain on oral antibiotics, with weekly checks undertaken until the foot shows clinical signs of stability. They are then placed into a moonboot with TTC insole, until custom footwear is available (**Table 16**).

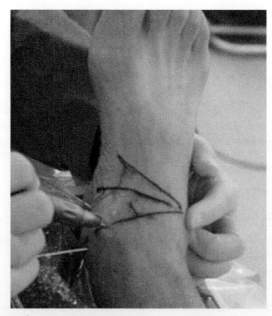

Fig. 8. Skin markings for osteotomy correction.

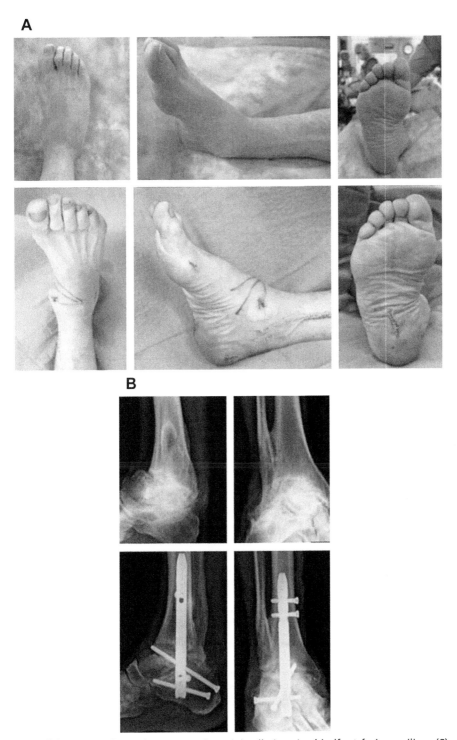

Fig. 9. (A) Preoperative and postoperative minimally invasive hindfoot fusion nailing. (B) Preoperative and postoperative minimally invasive hindfoot fusion nailing radiographs.

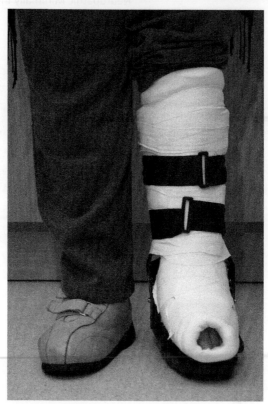

Fig. 10. Postoperative immobilization in an axial off-loader.

Table 16		
Outcomes at 2 years		
Forefoot	**Midfoot**	**Hindfoot**
5 debridement of osteomyelitis 4 lesser toe osteotomies to improve biomechanics Two 1st MTPJ arthrodesis 4 hallux valgus correction	14 midfoot fusions 4 with screws to the medial column TMT 6 with medium screws 2 infected medium bolts—removed and settled with antibiotics; foot position maintained and no reulceration	3 hindfoot fusion nails 3 debridement of calcaneal heel ulcers with prominent bone
1 digital amputation secondary to sepsis following debridement of osteomyelitis 1 recurrence of lesser toe deformity 1 recurrence of hallux valgus—revised to 1st MTPJ arthrodesis	2 medium screws failed as did not fully span the affected area—revised to long bolts 2 infected medium beams—requiring removal and repeated washout. Stable fibrous nonunion achieved with the foot remaining in the corrected position 1 breakage of metalwork. Stable fibrous union with the foot remaining in the corrected position	Fibrous nonunion of the ankle and subtalar joints, but remains stable and pain free Prominent heel screw which required removal
No re-ulceration No major amputations No deaths	No reulceration No major amputations No deaths	No reulceration No major amputations No deaths

SUMMARY

The initial results suggest that NEMISIS may offer potentially better surgical outcomes than traditional open surgical correction. There are complications associated with this type of surgery and postoperative management, but these can be anticipated, and with close supervision and the combined care of the multidisciplinary team, the major goals of prevention of reulceration, avoidance of major amputation, and death can be achieved.

Corrected foot positions can be maintained, despite subsequent removal of metalwork or fibrous nonunion. The surgery is dependent on access to good multidisciplinary clinical working to ensure the best outcomes and improve the quality and duration of life of the diabetic patient with foot abnormality.

NEMISIS may facilitate earlier stabilization, and therefore, shorten the treatment period and reduce the risk of amputation in this challenging patient group.

REFERENCES

1. NICE—Diabetic foot problems: preventions and management. NICE Guideline. 2015.
2. Armstrong DG, Wrobel J, Robbins JM. Guest editorial: are diabetes-related wounds and amputations worse than cancer. Int Wound J 2007;4:286–7.
3. International Diabetes Federation. IDF diabetes atlas. 7th edition. Brussels (Belgium): International Diabetes Federation; 2015. Available at: http://www.diabetesatlas.org/.
4. Rogers LC, Frykberg RG, Armstrong DG, et al. The Charcot foot. J Am Podiatr Med Assoc 2011;101:437–46.
5. Frykberg RG, Belczyk R. Epidemiology of the Charcot foot. Clin Podiatr Med Surg 2008;25:17–28.
6. Gregg EW, Sorlie P, Paulose-Ram R, et al. Prevalence of lower-extremity disease in the US adult population >=40 years of age with and without diabetes: 1999-2000 national health and nutrition examination survey. Diabetes Care 2004;27(7): 1591–7.
7. Lavery LA, Armstrong DG, Wunderlich RP, et al. Risk factors for foot infections in individuals with diabetes. Diabetes Care 2006;29(6):1288–93.
8. Pecoraro RE, Reiber GE, Burgess EM. Pathways to diabetic limb amputation. basis for prevention. Diabetes Care 1990;13(5):513–21.
9. Abbott CA, Carrington AL, Ashe H, et al. The North-West Diabetes Foot Care Study: incidence of, and risk factors for, new diabetic foot ulceration in a community-based patient cohort. Diabet Med 2002;19(5):377–84.
10. Boyko EJ, Ahroni JH, Cohen V, et al. Prediction of diabetic foot ulcer occurrence using commonly available clinical information: the Seattle Diabetic Foot Study. Diabetes Care 2006;29(6):1202–7.
11. Zimmet P. Globalization, coca-colonization and the chronic disease epidemic: can the doomsday scenario be averted? J Intern Med 2000;247:301–10.
12. Lauterbach S, Kostev K, Kohlmann T, et al. Prevalence of diabetic foot syndrome and its risk factors in the UK. J Wound Care 2010;19(8):333–7.
13. Zimmet PZ. Kelly West Lecture 1991. Challenges in diabetes epidemiology— from West to the rest. Diabetes Care 1992;15(2):232–52.
14. Subramaniam B, Pomposelli F, Talmor D, et al. Perioperative and long-term morbidity and mortality after above-knee and below-knee amputations in diabetics and nondiabetics. Anesth Analg 2005;100(5):1241–7.

15. McCabe CJ, Stevenson RC, Dolan AM. Evaluation of a diabetic foot screening and protection programme. Diabet Med 1998;15(1):80–4.

16. Gil J, Schiff AP, Pinzur MS. Cost comparison: limb salvage versus amputation in diabetic patients with Charcot foot. Foot Ankle Int 2013;34(8):1097–9.

17. Dalla Paola L. Confronting a dramatic situation: the Charcot foot complicated by osteomyelitis. Int J Low Extrem Wounds 2014;13(4):247–62.

18. Willrich A, Pinzur M, McNeil M, et al. Health related quality of life, cognitive function, and depression in diabetic patients with foot ulcer or amputation. A preliminary study. Foot Ankle Int 2005;26(2):128–34.

19. Pakarinen TK, Laine HJ, Maenpaa H, et al. Long-term outcome and quality of life in patients with Charcot foot. Foot Ankle Surg 2009;15:187–91.

20. Rogers LC, Frykberg RG, Armstrong DG, et al. The diabetic Charcot foot syndrome: a report of the Joint Task Force on the Charcot Foot by the American Diabetes Association and the American Podiatric Medical Association. Diabetes Care 2011;34:2123–9.

21. Gazis A, Pound N, Macfarlane R, et al. Mortality in patients with diabetic neuropathic osteoarthropathy (Charcot foot). Diabet Med 2004;21:1243–6.

22. Hansen ST, Pinzur MS. Debate: conservative, total contact casting vs. primary fusion of Charcot arthropathy of the foot. Specialty day meeting of the American Orthopaedic Foot and Ankle Society. New Orleans, February 08, 2003.

23. Pinzur MS, Evans A. Health related quality of life in patients with Charcot foot. Am J Orthop (Belle Mead NJ) 2003;32:492–6.

24. Saltzman CL, Domsic RT, Baumhauer JF, Deland JT, et al. Foot and ankle research priority: report from the Research Council of the American Orthopaedic Foot and Ankle Society. Foot Ankle Int 1997;18:443–6.

25. Schofield CJ, Libby G, Brennan GM, et al. Mortality and hospitalization in patients after amputation: a comparison between patients with and without diabetes. Diabetes Care 2006;29(10):2252–6.

26. Aulivola B, Hile CN, Hamdan HD, et al. Major lower extremity amputation: outcome of a modern series. Arch Surg 2004;139:395–9.

27. Pinzur MS, Gottschalk F, Smith D, et al. Functional outcome of below-knee amputation in peripheral vascular insufficiency. Clin Orthop 1993;286:247–9.

28. Izumi Y, Satterfield K, Lee S, et al. Mortality of first-time amputees in diabetics: a 10-year observation. Diabetes Res Clin Pract 2009;83(1):126–31.

29. Sohn MW, Lee TA, Stuck RM, et al. Mortality risk of Charcot arthropathy compared with that of diabetic foot ulcer and diabetes alone. Diabetes Care 2009;32(5):816–21.

30. Moulik PK, Mtonga R, Gill GV. Amputation and mortality in new-onset diabetic foot ulcers stratified by etiology. Diabetes Care 2003;26(2):491–4.

31. Lavery LA, Peters EJ, Armstrong DG, et al. Risk factors for developing osteomyelitis in patients with diabetic foot wounds. Diabetes Res Clin Pract 2009;83(3):347–52.

32. Agency for Healthcare Research and Quality, Rockville, MD. Type 2 Diabetes. October 2014. Available at: http://www.ahrq.gov/professionals/education/curriculum-tools/diabnotebk/diabnotebk23.html.

33. Stone PA, Flaherty SK, Hayes JD, et al. Lower extremity amputation: a contemporary series. W V Med J 2007;103(5):14–8.

34. Peters EJ, Lavery LA, International Working Group on the Diabetic Foot. Effectiveness of the diabetic foot risk classification system of the International Working Group on the Diabetic Foot. Diabetes Care 2001;24(8):1442–7.

35. Margolis DJ, Allen-Taylor L, Hoffstad O, et al. Diabetic neuropathic foot ulcers and amputation. Wound Repair Regen 2005;13(3):230–6.
36. Sohn M-W, Stuck RM, Pinzur M, et al. Lower-extremity amputation risk after Charcot arthropathy and diabetic foot ulcer. Diabetes Care 2010;33(1):98–100.
37. Pinzur MS. Benchmark analysis of diabetic patients with neuropathic (Charcot) foot deformity. Foot Ankle Int 1999;20:564–7.
38. Saltzman CL, Hagy ML, Zimmerman B, et al. How effective is intensive nonoperative initial treatment of patients with diabetes and Charcot arthropathy of the feet? Clin Orthop Relat Res 2005;435:185–90.
39. Reiber GE, Vileikyte L, Boyko EJ, et al. Causal pathways for incident lower-extremity ulcers in patients with diabetes from two settings. Diabetes Care 1999;22(1):157–62.
40. O'Neal L. The diabetic foot. 7th edition. Maryland Heights (MO): Mosby; 2008. p. 24, 31, 34, 190–2, 350–1, 405.
41. Trautman JR, Kirchheimer WF, Prabhakaran K, et al. An overview of Carville research. Acta Leprol 1981;(84):1–29.
42. Nazimek-Siewniak B, Moczulski D, Grzeszczak W. Risk of macrovascular and microvascular complications in type 2 diabetes: results of longitudinal study design. J Diabet Complications 2002;16:271–6.
43. Mabilleau G, Petrova NL, Edmonds ME, et al. Increased osteoclastic activity in acute Charcot arthropathy: the role of receptor activator of nuclear factor-kappaB Ligand. Diabetologia 2008;51:1035–40.
44. Bessman AN, Sapico FL. Infections in the diabetic patient: the role of immune dysfunction and pathogen virulence factors. J Diabet Complications 1992;6: 258–62.
45. Bergtholdt HT, Brand PW. Thermography: an aid in the management of insensitive feet and stumps. Arch Phys Med Rehabil 1975;56:205–9.
46. Young MJ, Cavanagh PR, Thomas G, et al. The effect of callus removal on dynamic plantar foot pressures in diabetic patients. Diabet Med 1992;9:55–7.
47. Grant WP, Sullivan R, Sonenshine DE, et al. Electron microscopic investigation of the effects of diabetes mellitus on the Achilles tendon. J Foot Ankle Surg 1997; 36(4):272–8 [discussion: 330].
48. Reddy GK. Cross-linking in collagen by nonenzymatic glycation increases the matrix stiffness in rabbit Achilles tendon. Exp Diabesity Res 2004;5(2):143–53.
49. Reddy GK. Glucose-mediated in vitro glycation modulates biomechanical integrity of the soft tissues but not hard tissues. J Orthop Res 2003;21(4):738–43.
50. Mueller MJ, Sinacore DR, Hastings MK, et al. Effect of Achilles tendon lengthening on neuropathic plantar ulcers. A randomized clinical trial. J Bone Joint Surg Am 2003;85:1436–45.
51. Jeffcoate WJ, Game FL. New theories on the causes of the Charcot foot in diabetes. In: Frykberg RG, editor. The diabetic Charcot foot: principles and management. Brooklandville (MD): Data Trace Publishing Company; 2010. p. 29–44.
52. Jeffcoate WJ, Game F, Cavanagh PR. The role of proinflammatory cytokines in the cause of neuropathic osteoarthropathy (acute Charcot foot) in diabetes. Lancet 2005;366:2058–61.
53. Falanga V. Wound healing and its impairment in the diabetic foot. Lancet 2005; 366:1736–43.
54. Stojadinovic O, Brem H, Vouthounis C, et al. Molecular pathogenesis of chronic wounds: the role of beta-catenin and c-myc in the inhibition of epithelialization and wound healing. Am J Pathol 2005;167:59–69.

55. Dorweiler B, Neufang A, Kreitner KF, et al. Magnetic resonance angiography unmasks reliable target vessels for pedal bypass grafting in patients with diabetes mellitus. J Vasc Surg 2002;35:766–72.

56. Rogers LC, Bevilacqua N. Imaging of the Charcot foot. Clin Podiatr Med Surg 2008;25:263–74.

57. Tan PL, Teh J. MRI of the diabetic foot: differentiation of infection from neuropathic change. Br J Radiol 2007;80:939–48.

58. Herbst SA, Jones KB, Saltzman CL. Pattern of diabetic neuropathic arthropathy associated with the peripheral bone mineral density. J Bone Joint Surg Br 2004; 86:378–83.

59. Newman JH. Non-infective disease of the diabetic foot. J Bone Joint Surg Br 1981;63:593–6.

60. Garapati R, Weinfeld SB. Complex reconstruction of the diabetic foot and ankle. Am J Surg 2004;187(5A):81S–6S.

61. Rajbhandari SM, Jenkins RC, Davies C, et al. Charcot neuroarthropathy in diabetes mellitus. Diabetologia 2002;45:1085–96.

62. Eichenholtz SN. Charcot joints. Springfield (IL): Charles C Thomas; 1966.

63. Schon LC, Easley ME, Cohen I, et al. The acquired midtarsus deformity classification system-interobserver reliability and intraobserver reproducibility. Foot Ankle Int 2015;23(1):1–7.

64. Shibata T, Tada K, Hashizume C. The result of arthrodesis of the ankle for leprotic neuroarthropathy. J Bone Joint Surg Am 1990;72:749–56.

65. Schon LC, Easley ME, Weinfeld SB. Charcot neuroarthropathy of the foot and ankle. Clin Orthop 1998;349:116–31.

66. Wukich DK, Raspovic KM, Hobizal KB, et al. Radiographic analysis of diabetic midfoot Charcot neuroarthropathy with and without midfoot ulceration. Foot Ankle Int 2014;35(11):1108–15.

67. Pellizzer G, Strazzabosco M, Presi S, et al. Deep tissue biopsy vs. superficial swab culture monitoring in the microbiological assessment of limb-threatening diabetic foot infection. Diabet Med 2001;18:822–7.

68. Kessler L, Piemont Y, Ortega F, et al. Comparison of microbiological results of needle puncture vs. superficial swab in infected diabetic foot ulcer with osteomyelitis. Diabet Med 2006;23:99–102.

69. Selia EJ, Barette C. Staging of Charcot neuroarthropathy along the medial column of the foot in the diabetic patient. J Foot Ankle Surg 1999;38(1):34–40.

70. Senneville E, Melliez H, Beltrand E, et al. Culture of percutaneous bone biopsy specimens for diagnosis of diabetic foot osteomyelitis: concordance with ulcer swab cultures. Clin Infect Dis 2006;42:57–62.

71. Pinzur M. Surgical versus accommodative treatment for Charcot arthropathy of the midfoot. Foot Ankle Int 2004;25(8):545–9.

72. Ha Van G, Siney H, Hartmann-Heurtier A, et al. Nonremovable, windowed, fiberglass cast boot in the treatment of diabetic plantar ulcers: efficacy, safety, and compliance. Diabetes Care 2003;26:2848–52.

73. Pinzur MS, Sage R, Stuck R, et al. Treatment algorithm for neuropathic (Charcot) midfoot deformity. Foot Ankle Int 1993;14:189–97.

74. Wu SC, Jensen JL, Weber AK, et al. Use of pressure offloading devices in diabetic foot ulcers: do we practice what we preach? Diabetes Care 2008;31: 2118–9.

75. Boulton AJ, Bowker JH, Gadia M, et al. Use of plaster casts in the management of diabetic neuropathic foot ulcers. Diabetes Care 1986;9:149–52.

76. Praet SF, Louwerens JW. The influence of shoe design on plantar pressures in neuropathic feet. Diabetes Care 2003;26:441–5.
77. Mueller MJ, Strube MJ, Allen BT. Therapeutic footwear can reduce plantar pressures in patients with diabetes and transmetatarsal amputation. Diabetes Care 1997;20:637–41.
78. Osterhoff G, Böni T, Berli M. Recurrence of acute Charcot neuropathic osteoarthropathy after conservative treatment. Foot Ankle Int 2013;34(3):359–64.
79. Apelqvist J, Larsson J, Agardh CD. Long-term prognosis for diabetic patients with foot ulcers. J Intern Med 1993;233(6):485–91.
80. Lind J, Kramhoft M, Bodtker S. The influence of smoking on complications after primary amputations of the lower extremity. Clin Orthop Relat Res 1991;(267):211–7.
81. Crim BE, Wukich DK. Osteomyelitis of the foot and ankle in the diabetic population: diagnosis and treatment. J Diabet Foot Complications 2010;1:25–35.
82. Arad Y, Fonseca V, Peters A, et al. Beyond the monofilament for the insensate diabetic foot: a systematic review of randomized trials to prevent the occurrence of plantar foot ulcers in patients with diabetes. Diabetes Care 2011;34:1041–6.
83. Armstrong DG, Lavery LA. Monitoring healing of acute Charcot's arthropathy with infrared dermal thermometry. J Rehabil Res Dev 1997;34:317–21.
84. Ge Y, MacDonald D, Hait H, et al. Microbiological profile of infected diabetic foot ulcers. Diabet Med 2002;19:1032–4.
85. Lowery NJ, Woods JB, Armstrong DG, et al. Surgical management of Charcot neuroarthropathy of the foot and ankle: a systematic review. Foot Ankle Int 2012;33(02):113 21.
86. Pinzur MS. Neutral ring fixation for high-risk nonplantigrade Charcot midfoot deformity. Foot Ankle Int 2007;28:961–6.
87. Pinzur MS, Sostak J. Surgical stabilization of nonplantigrade Charcot arthropathy of the midfoot. Am J Orthop 2007;36:361–5.
88. Papa J, Myerson M, Girard P. Salvage, with arthrodeses, in intractable diabetic neuropathic arthropathy of the foot and ankle. J Bone Joint Surg Am 1993;75:1056–66.
89. Sammarco GJ, Conti SF. Surgical treatment of neuroarthropathic foot deformity. Foot Ankle Int 1998;19:102–9.
90. Mittlmeier T, Klaue K, Haar P, et al. Should one consider primary surgical reconstruction in Charcot arthropathy of the feet? Clin Orthop Relat Res 2010;468(4):1002–11.
91. Schade CP, Hannah KL. Quality of ambulatory care for diabetes and lower-extremity amputation. Am J Med Qual 2007;22(6):410–7.
92. Bevilacqua NJ, Rogers LC, Armstrong DG. Diabetic foot surgery: classifying patients to predict complications. Diabetes Metab Res Rev 2008;24(Suppl 1):S81–3.
93. Clohisy DR, Thompson RC Jr. Fractures associated with neuropathic arthropathy in adults who have juvenile-onset diabetes. J Bone Joint Surg Am 1988;70:1192–200.
94. Sammarco VJ, Sammarco GJ, Walker EW Jr, et al. Mid-tarsal arthrodesis in the treatment of Charcot midfoot arthropathy. J Bone Joint Surg Am 2009;91:80–91.
95. Greenhagen RM, Johnson AR, Peterson MC, et al. Gastrocnemius recession as an alternative to tendoAchillis lengthening for relief of forefoot pressure in a patient with peripheral neuropathy: a case report and description of a technical modification. J Foot Ankle Surg 2010;49:159.e9-e13.

96. Laborde JM. Tendon lengthening for neuropathic foot problems. Orthopedics 2010;33:319–26.
97. Laborde JM. Treatment of diabetic foot ulcers with tendon lengthening. Am Fam Physician 2009;80:1351 [author reply: 1351].
98. Tamir E, McLaren AM, Gadgil A, et al. Outpatient percutaneous flexor tenotomies for management of diabetic claw toe deformities with ulcers: a preliminary report. Can J Surg 2008;51:41–4.
99. Brodsky JW, Rouse AM. Esostectomy for symptomatic bony prominences in diabetic Charcot feet. Clin Orthop Relat Res 1993;296:21–6.
100. Pope E, Takemoto RC, Kummer FJ, et al. Midfoot fusion:a biomechanical comparison of plantar planting vs intramedullary screws. Foot Ankle Int 2015;34(3): 409–13.
101. Conway JD. Charcot salvage of the foot and ankle using external fixation. Foot Ankle Clin 2008;13:157–73.
102. Zarutsky E, Rush SM, Schuberth JM. The use of circular wire external fixation in the treatment of salvage ankle arthrodesis. J Foot Ankle Surg 2005;44:22–31.
103. Van Der Ven A, Chapman CB, Bowker JH. Charcot neuroarthropathy of the foot and ankle. J Am Acad Orthop Surg 2009;17:562–71.
104. Lamm BM, Gottlieb HD, Paley D. A two-stage percutaneous approach to Charcot diabetic foot reconstruction. J Foot Ankle Surg 2010;49:517–22.
105. Sammarco VJ. Superconstructs in the treatment of Charcot foot deformity: plantar plating, locked plating, and axial screw fixation. Foot Ankle Clin 2009; 14:393–407.
106. Grant WP, Garcia-Lavin S, Sabo R. Beaming the columns for Charcot diabetic foot reconstruction: a retrospective analysis. J Foot Ankle Surg 2011;50:182–9.
107. Grant WP. Biomechanics of the Charcot foot collapse and riding the medial column of the foot as a beam to salvage the Charcot foot. Paper presented at: Annual American College of Foot and Ankle Surgeons Scientific Seminar. Orlando, February 5–8, 1997.
108. Norkin CC, Levangie PK. Joint structure & function: a comprehensive analysis. Philadelphia: F A Davies Company; 1992. p. 2, 379–415.
109. Harris JR, Brand PW. Patterns of disintegration of the tarsus in the anesthetic foot. J Bone Joint Surg Br 1966;48B(1):4–16.
110. Pell RF, Myerson MS, Schon LC. Clinical outcome after primary triple arthrodesis. J Bone Joint Surg Am 2000;82-A:47–57.
111. Simon SR, Tejwani SG, Wilson DL, et al. Arthrodesis as an early alternative to nonoperative management of Charcot arthropathy of the diabetic foot. J Bone Joint Surg Am 2000;82:939–50.
112. Baravarian B, Van Gils CC. Arthrodesis of the Charcot foot and ankle. Clin Podiatr Med Surg 2004;21:271–89.
113. Early JS, Hansen ST. Surgical reconstruction of the diabetic foot: a salvage approach for midfoot collapse. Foot Ankle Int 1996;17:325–30.
114. Marks RM, Parks BG, Schon LC. Midfoot fusion technique for neuropathic feet: biomechanical analysis and rationale. Foot Ankle Int 1998;19:507–10.
115. Myerson MS, Alvarez RG, Lam PW. Tibiocalcaneal arthrodesis for the management of severe ankle and hindfoot deformities. Foot Ankle Int 2000;21:643–50.
116. Brem H, Sheehan P, Rosenberg HJ, et al. Evidence-based protocol for diabetic foot ulcers. Plast Reconstr Surg 2006;117(Suppl 7):193S–209S.
117. Attinger CE, Ducic I, Cooper P, et al. The role of intrinsic muscle flaps of the foot for bone coverage in foot and ankle defects in diabetic and nondiabetic patients. Plast Reconstr Surg 2002;110:1047–54.

118. Bong MR, Kummer FJ, Koval KJ, et al. Intramedullary nailing of the lower extremity biomechanics and biology. J Am Acad Orthop Surg 2007;15(2): 97–106.

119. Kessler SB, Hallfeldt KKJ, Perren SM, et al. The effects of reaming and intramedullary nailing on fracture healing. Clin Orthop Relat Res 1986;(212):18–25.

120. Chapman MW. The effect of reamed and nonreamed intramedullary nailing on fracture healing. Clin Orthop Relat Res 1998;(Suppl 355):S230–8.

121. Bhandari M, Guyatt GH, Tong D, et al. Reamed versus non- reamed intramedullary nailing of lower extremity long bone fractures: a systemic overview and meta-analysis. J Orthop Trauma 2000;14(1):2–9.

Percutaneous Hindfoot and Midfoot Fusion

Thomas Bauer, MD, PhD

KEYWORDS

- Percutaneous foot surgery • Ankle fusion • Subtalar fusion • Triple fusion

KEY POINTS

- Hindfoot and midfoot fusions can be performed with percutaneous techniques.
- Preliminary results of these procedures are encouraging because they provide similar results than those obtained with open techniques with less morbidity and quick recovery.
- The best indications are probably fusions for mild-to-moderate reducible hindfoot and midfoot deformities in fragile patients with general or local bad conditions.
- The main limit is linked to the surgeon's experience in percutaneous foot surgery because a learning curve with the specific tools is necessary before doing these procedures.

INTRODUCTION

Open hindfoot and midfoot fusions are associated with a high rate of complications (around 20%), including nonunions, infections, wound dehiscence, and scar problems.[1,2] These complications can be avoided with an arthroscopic or minimally invasive approach that theoretically prevents skin problems.[3–6] Percutaneous techniques are now well-established procedures in forefoot surgery but are less frequently performed for hindfoot and midfoot abnormalities. The goals of performing hindfoot and midfoot fusions with percutaneous techniques are to obtain results at least as good as open techniques with a quicker recovery and fewer risks of complications for the patient.

INDICATIONS/CONTRAINDICATIONS

Indications for performing hindfoot and midfoot fusions with percutaneous technique are basically the same as those with open and conventional techniques:

- Tibiotalar osteoarthritis (posttraumatic, idiopathic)
- Subtalar osteoarthritis (posttraumatic, idiopathic)
- Midtarsal osteoarthritis (posttraumatic, idiopathic)

Dr Bauber is a paid consultant for Arthrex.
Department of Orthopedic Surgery, Ambroise Paré Hospital, West Paris University, 9 Avenue Charles de Gaulle, Boulogne 92100, France
E-mail address: thomas.bauer@aphp.fr

Foot Ankle Clin N Am 21 (2016) 629–640
http://dx.doi.org/10.1016/j.fcl.2016.04.008
1083-7515/16/$ – see front matter © 2016 Elsevier Inc. All rights reserved.

foot.theclinics.com

- Tibiotalar, subtalar, and midtarsal arthritis (rheumatoid arthritis, inflammatory arthritis, septic arthritis)
- Mild-to-moderate deformities: hindfoot valgus, pes planus, cavovarus deformity.

It makes sense to propose percutaneous hindfoot and midfoot fusions for patients with local or general bad conditions (skin problems, previous scars, arteriopathy, diabetes, immunodeficiency, elderly people) because they are at higher risk of complication with open procedures.

There are basically 2 main contraindications:

- Anatomic contraindication: for severe and fixed deformities or severe bone loss (requiring bone graft), the percutaneous procedure might be more difficult and time consuming regarding the joint surfaces preparation and reliability of fusion.
- Contraindication linked to the surgeon's experience: depending on the experience of each surgeon in percutaneous foot procedures, some situations might be considered as relative contraindications for percutaneous fusion.

TIBIOTALAR FUSION
Preoperative Planning

Percutaneous ankle fusion may be challenging in the case of fixed and severe deformities with bone loss. Preoperative clinical assessment is essential to assess the reducibility of the deformities (hindfoot varus or valgus, equinus). Reducible and mild-to-moderate deformities are good situations to propose ankle fusion with a percutaneous technique. Iconographic assessment with radiographs and computed tomographic (CT) scan are useful to assess tibiotalar subluxation, bone loss, and tibial or talar osteophytes. Tibiotalar subluxation (most often anterior) is a difficult situation because the reduction of the talus under the tibial plafond is necessary to get an optimal position for the ankle fusion. This reduction is often difficult to obtain with a percutaneous (or arthroscopic) technique. Lateral view on the radiographs can show anterior osteophytes that can close the anterior space and prevent access to the ankle joint line (**Fig. 1**). It is important to know preoperatively if some osteophytes have to be removed before preparing the joint surfaces and to adapt the portals depending on the position and size of these osteophytes.

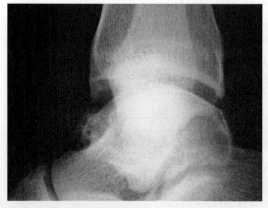

Fig. 1. Anterior prominent tibotalar osteophytes on lateral view.

Patient Positioning

The patient is settled in the supine position with the foot and ankle free at the end of the table. A support is placed under the ipsilateral buttock to have the foot vertical. A tourniquet can be used and placed on the thigh. A mini C-arm is placed at the end of the table for fluoroscopic control with anteroposterior (AP) and lateral views.

Surgical Approach

Two main portals are used: one anteromedial portal medial to the tibialis anterior tendon (the same anteromedial portal as used for anterior ankle arthroscopy) and one anterolateral portal (at the level of the lateral corner of the tibiotalar joint line) (**Fig. 2**). Two accessory portals may be used: one medial at the tip of the medial malleolus and one lateral at the tip of the lateral malleolus (**Fig. 3**).

Surgical Procedure

The first step is the removal of the osteophytes and cartilage of the tibiotalar joint. A 5-mm incision is made at the anteromedial and anterolateral portal. A conical 4-mm burr is used and inserted in the tibiotalar joint space alternatively through the anteromedial and anterolateral portal (**Fig. 4**). In the case of prominent anterior osteophyte, the first step is to remove it with the burr before accessing the ankle joint. Fluoroscopic control with AP and lateral views confirms the good position of the burr on the osteophyte and at the level of the ankle joint line. Cartilage removal begins from anterior to posterior (**Fig. 5**). The burr is progressively pushed posteriorly by opening the ankle joint space with distraction and plantar flexion if needed. Cartilage debris is carefully removed with rasps and curettes, and the tibiotalar space is abundantly cleaned with saline (**Fig. 6**).

The second step is the removal of the osteophytes and cartilage of the malleolar grooves (see **Fig. 6**B; **Fig. 7**A). Through the anteromedial portal, the burr is pushed distally in the medial malleolar groove to remove the talar and malleolar cartilage and the osteophytes. It is sometimes necessary to use an accessory medial portal

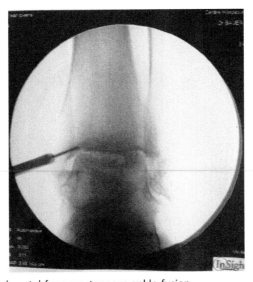

Fig. 2. Anteromedial portal for percutaneous ankle fusion.

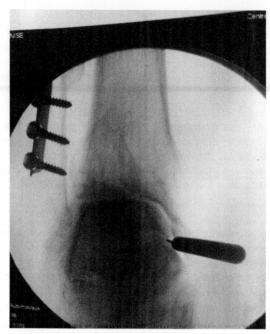

Fig. 3. Accessory anteromedial portal for percutaneous ankle fusion.

at the tip of the medial malleolus to enable better removal of cartilage and obtain complete release of the medial malleolar groove. The lateral malleolar groove is then prepared with the same technique through the anterolateral portal and the accessory lateral portal to access the tip of the lateral malleolus and remove the cartilage of the lateral talar facet. Cartilage debris is carefully removed with rasps and curettes, and the tibiotalar space is abundantly cleaned with saline.

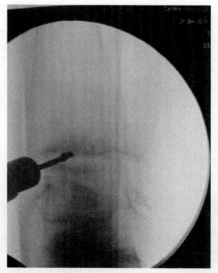

Fig. 4. Removal of the tibiotalar cartilage with the burr in the anteromedial portal.

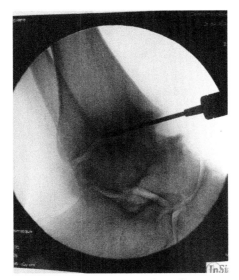

Fig. 5. Removal of the tibiotalar cartilage with the burr: fluoroscopic control.

The third step is the bone surfaces preparation. A fluoroscopic AP and lateral view are performed with the ankle maintained in a 90° position with the hindfoot aligned and compression to assess the quality of the bone preparation (bone contact, position of the talus under the tibia). In the case of remnant radiolucency at the level of the joint line, additional removal of cartilage and subchondral bone is performed with curettes and burr to obtain a complete bony contact between the talus and the tibia.

The fourth step is the fixation of the ankle fusion. Compression is applied on the ankle in a 90° position with good alignment of the hindfoot confirmed on the fluoroscopic control. Three pins (2 tibiotalar and 1 fibulotalar) are placed, and their position is assessed on AP and lateral views (**Fig. 8**). Then,

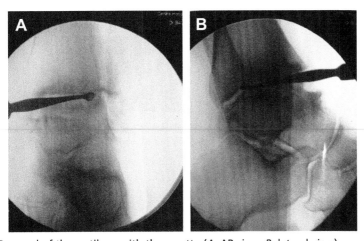

Fig. 6. Removal of the cartilage with the curette (*A*: AP view; *B*: lateral view).

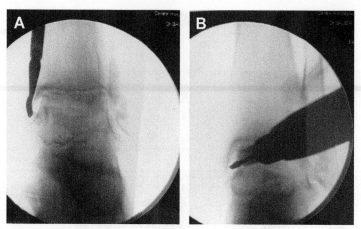

Fig. 7. Preparation of the medial malleolar gutter (*A*: release with an elevator; *B*: removal of the cartilage of the medial gutter with the burr).

6- or 7-mm cannulated screws are inserted to make the final fixation and give compression.

SUBTALAR FUSION
Preoperative Planning

The main difficulty when performing percutaneous subtalar fusion is to obtain good hindfoot alignment. Clinical preoperative planning must assess hindfoot malalignment (varus or valgus) and the reducibility of the deformity. Reducible deformities are good situations to perform subtalar fusion with percutaneous technique. Iconographic preoperative planning (radiographs and CT scan) must assess any bone loss on the talar

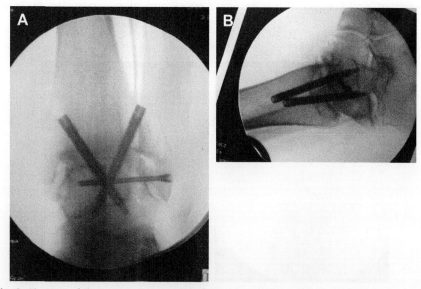

Fig. 8. Fixation of the percutaneous ankle fusion (*A*: AP view; *B*: lateral view).

or calcaneal side. Reducible and mild-to-moderate hindfoot deformities without major bone loss are good conditions to perform subtalar fusion with percutaneous technique.

Patient Positioning

The patient is settled in the lateral position with the foot and ankle free at the end of the table. A tourniquet can be used and placed on the thigh. A mini C-arm is placed at the end of the table for the fluoroscopic control with AP and lateral views.

Surgical Approach

One main anterolateral portal is used to perform percutaneous subtalar fusion: the portal is located at the sinus tarsi (1 cm distal and 1.5 cm anterior to the tip of the lateral malleolus).

Surgical Procedure

The first step is the removal of the cartilage of the subtalar joint. A 5-mm incision is made at the sinus tarsi location to create the anterolateral portal. Elevators are then inserted into the sinus tarsi and in the posterior part of the subtalar joint line. A conical 4-mm burr is used and inserted in the subtalar joint line through the anterolateral portal. Cartilage removal begins from anterior and lateral to posterior. The burr is progressively pushed medially by opening the lateral subtalar space with the other hand creating distraction and slight hindfoot varus. Cartilage debris is carefully removed with rasps and curettes, and the subtalar space is abundantly cleaned with saline (**Fig. 9A**).

The second step is the bone surface preparation. Hindfoot compression in a straight position is applied, and a fluoroscopic control is then performed with a lateral view to assess the quality of the bone preparation (bone contact, position of the subtalar facets). In the case of remnant joint space on the lateral view, additional removal of cartilage and subchondral bone is performed with curettes and burr to obtain a flat bone surface without remnant radiolucency on lateral view.

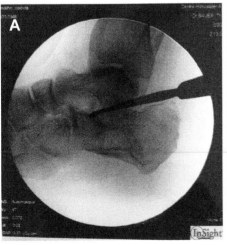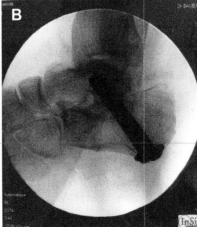

Fig. 9. Percutaneous subtalar fusion (*A*: removal of the cartilage with a curette; *B*: fixation with 2 cannulated screws).

The third step is the fixation of the subtalar fusion. The position of the hindfoot is maintained with one hand to keep compression of the subtalar joint and alignment of the hindfoot, and 2 calcaneotalar pins are inserted from the heel with the other hand. Fluoroscopic control (with AP and lateral view) is then made to assess the good position of the pins, the quality of the subtalar position, and compression. Then, 2 cannulated 6- or 7-mm screws are inserted for the fixation of the subtalar fusion (**Fig. 9**B).

TRIPLE FUSION
Preoperative Planning

Triple fusion is mostly indicated for painful pes planus or cavo varus deformities with osteoarthritic changes. The main difficulty of performing a triple fusion with a percutaneous technique is linked to the reducibility of the deformity. Severe and stiff deformities will be difficult cases for a percutaneous procedure because the possibility of reduction remains limited. The clinical preoperative planning will focus on the reducibility of the deformity, making it a good indication for a percutaneous procedure. Radiological preoperative planning is essential to assess any bone loss (most frequently on the navicular bone) that would require a bone graft and will represent a contraindication for a percutaneous procedure.

Patient Positioning

The patient is settled in semilateral position with the foot and ankle free at the end of the table. A tourniquet can be used and placed on the thigh. A mini C-arm is placed at the end of the table for the fluoroscopic control with AP and lateral views.

Surgical Approach

Percutaneous triple fusion can be performed with 3 portals:

- One subtalar portal (the same used for the percutaneous subtalar fusion)
- One calcaneocuboid portal: lateral, at the level of the calcaneocuboid joint line
- One talonavicular portal: dorsomedial, at the level of the talonavicular joint line, medial from the tibialis anterior tendon. Sometimes, depending on the severity of the deformity or on the access of the talonavicular joint (especially its plantar part), an accessory medial portal can be done on the medial facet of the talonavicular joint, just dorsal from the tibialis posterior tendon.

Surgical Procedure

The first step is the preparation the subtalar joint with the same technique described for percutaneous subtalar fusion (**Fig. 10**A, B).

The second step is the calcaneocuboid joint preparation. Through the lateral portal, the burr is inserted into the calcaneocuboid joint space to remove all the cartilage (**Fig. 10**C). A fluoroscopic lateral view confirms the complete removal of the cartilage and good bone contact. Cartilage debris is carefully removed with rasps and curettes, and the subtalar space is abundantly cleaned with saline.

The third step is talonavicular joint preparation. Cartilage is removed with the burr through the dorsomedial portal (**Fig. 10**D). Fluoroscopic control (with AP and lateral view) is necessary to assess the quality of cartilage removal, reduction of the talonavicular joint, and necessity of performing an additional medial portal to have a complete preparation.

The final step is the reduction of the deformities (starting with subtalar joint and ending with the midtarsal joint) and fixation. Percutaneous subtalar joint fusion is

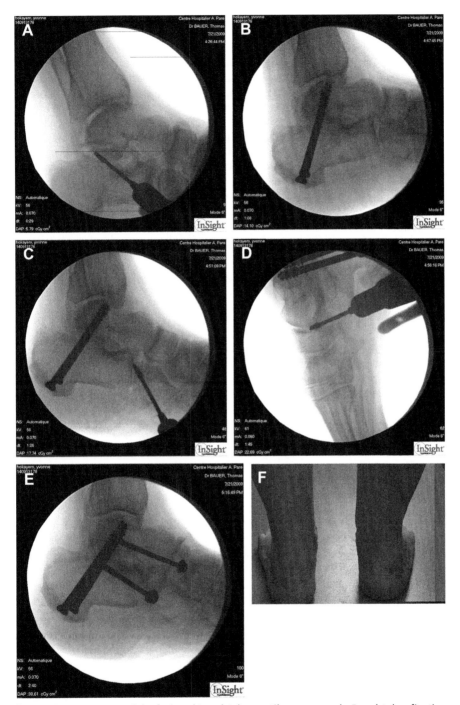

Fig. 10. Percutaneous triple fusion (*A*: subtalar cartilage removal; *B*: subtalar fixation; *C*: calcaneocuboid preparation; *D*: talonavicular preparation; *E*: radiological aspect at 2 months; *F*: clinical aspect at 2 months, right foot).

performed with the same technique as described earlier. Fluoroscopic control with AP and lateral view is necessary to assess the quality of bone contact, the hindfoot alignment, the restoration of talar height on the calcaneus, and the reduction of the talocalcaneal angle. The subtalar fusion can be fixed with one or two 6- or 7-mm cannulated screws. After subtalar fixation, the midtarsal correction is performed, acting simultaneously on midfoot abduction/adduction, medial arch restoration, and forefoot pronation/supination. Depending on the reducibility of the deformities, the fixation can be started on the calcaneocuboid joint or on the talonavicular joint. When the desired correction is obtained and fluoroscopic control confirms the good position of the midtarsal joints and good bone contact, the fixation is performed with 4-mm cannulated screws. One calcaneocuboid screw and 1 or 2 talonavicular screws are necessary for the fixation (**Fig. 10**E, F).

POSTOPERATIVE CARE

After percutaneous tibiotalar fusion and triple fusion, patients are immobilized in a cast without weight-bearing for the first 6 weeks. Progressive full weight-bearing is begun after 6 weeks.

After isolated percutaneous subtalar fusion, patients are immobilized with an ankle brace with immediate full weight-bearing as tolerated.

COMPLICATIONS AND MANAGEMENT

The first difficulty of percutaneous hindfoot and midfoot fusions is the management of the portals that must be chosen clinically by palpation and mobilization to have a direct access to the joints. Prominent tibiotalar osteophytes may prevent access of the ankle joint and can lead to displaced portals in relation to the level of the joint line. In these situations, a preoperative fluoroscopic control is necessary to check the positioning of the portals for both osteophyte removal and joint surfaces preparation.

Depending on the subchondral bone density, preparation of the surfaces may be difficult with inadequate cartilage removal on sclerotic areas and bone loss on soft areas. These technical difficulties will lead to inhomogeneous surface preparation with risks of remaining deformities and nonunions. It is thus important to check preoperatively on the radiographs the location of any sclerotic areas where the preparation with the burr will be more difficult (with risk of heat of the drill and bone or soft tissues burns). On the other hand, the burr must be handled smoothly on soft areas to avoid excessive bone loss. These sensations with the burr are very important to have a safe procedure without excessive fluoroscopic control. It is thus obvious that experience in percutaneous surgery with the specific tools is mandatory before beginning with hindfoot and midfoot percutaneous fusions.

Some pitfalls are specific for each type of procedure.

- For the percutaneous ankle fusion, the main risk is inadequate cartilage removal and bone or skin burn due to sclerotic bone (on talar dome and tibial plafond) and osteophytes, making the work difficult with heat of the burr and drill. Asymmetric surface preparation can occur with too much resection on the anterior part of the tibiotalar space and risk of unstable fixation or anterior subluxation of the talus. Distraction with progressive plantar flexion of the ankle is necessary to avoid this risk.
- For the percutaneous subtalar fusion, the main risk is asymmetric surface preparation with too much bone resection on the lateral part of the subtalar joint, increasing the risk of residual excessive hindfoot valgus. Distraction during the

removal of the cartilage with the burr and progressive resection from lateral to medial avoid this complication.

- For the percutaneous triple fusion, the main risk of the calcaneocuboid joint preparation is excessive bone resection (as the surfaces are often soft) with shortening of the lateral column during compression on the calcaneocuboid joint and residual midfoot abduction. To avoid this bone loss on the calcaneocuboid joint, it can be useful to insert a mosquito clamp in the joint as an internal distractor and to resect more on the medial part than on the lateral part in order to keep a stable and strong lateral cortex without excessive shortening. The talonavicular joint is probably the more difficult to prepare with the burr because of the anatomy of the joint (curved surfaces, deep part of the navicular bone) and because of the difference of bone density between the talar head (soft bone) and the navicular (hard and sclerotic bone). The preparation with the burr is thus difficult with a risk of insufficient surface preparation on the navicular side and bone loss on the talar side. Progressive fluoroscopic controls during cartilage removal are necessary to keep safe and efficient work.

OUTCOMES

The clinical mid-term and long-term results of these percutaneous hindfoot and midfoot fusions are basically similar to those obtained with conventional open or arthroscopic procedures. The 2 main advantages of these percutaneous procedures are

- The decreased postoperative pain and hospital stay (these procedures can be performed on outpatients)
- The decreased morbidity with less wound and septic complications.

Compared with arthroscopic-assisted hindfoot fusions, percutaneous procedures are less operative time consuming.[3–6] These percutaneous procedures are thus very interesting for fragile patients or patients with local bad conditions because they provide a functional improvement with a quick recovery and less risk.

SUMMARY

Hindfoot and midfoot fusions can be performed with percutaneous techniques. Preliminary results of these procedures are encouraging because they provide similar results than those obtained with open techniques with less morbidity and quick recovery. The best indications are probably fusions for mild-to-moderate reducible hindfoot and midfoot deformities in fragile patients with general or local bad conditions. The main limit is linked to the surgeon's experience in percutaneous foot surgery because a learning curve with the specific tools is necessary before doing these procedures.

REFERENCES

1. Frey C, Halikus NM, Vu-Rose T, et al. A review of ankle arthrodesis: predisposing factors to nonunion. Foot Ankle Int 1994;15(11):581–4.
2. Helm R. The results of ankle arthrodesis. J Bone Joint Surg Br 1990;72:141–3.
3. Glick JM, Morgan CD, Myerson MS, et al. Ankle arthrodesis using an arthroscopic method: long-term follow-up of 34 cases. Arthroscopy 1996;12(4):428–34.
4. Kats J, van Kampen A, de Waal-Malefijt MC. Improvement in technique for arthroscopic ankle fusion: results in 15 patients. Knee Surg Sports Traumatol Arthrosc 2003;11(1):46–9.

5. Raikin SM. Arthrodesis of the ankle: arthroscopic, mini-open, and open techniques. Foot Ankle Clin 2003;8(2):347–59.
6. Carranza-Bencano A, Tejero-Garcia S, Del Castillo-Blanco G, et al. Isolated subtalar arthrodesis through minimal incision surgery. Foot Ankle Int 2013;34(8): 1117–27.

A Proposed Staging Classification for Minimally Invasive Management of Haglund's Syndrome with Percutaneous and Endoscopic Surgery

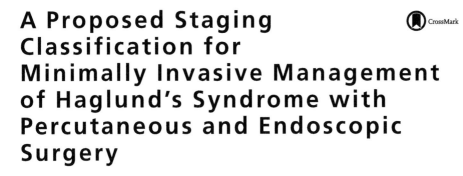

Turab Arshad Syed, MBBS, MRCS (GB), MFSEM (UK), DipSICOT, FRCS Eng (Tr& Orth), MSc (Bath)*,
Anthony Perera, MBChB, MRCS, MFSEM, PG Dip(Med Law), FRCS (Orth)

KEYWORDS

- Haglund's syndrome • Achilles tendonopathy • Minimally invasive approach
- Endoscopy • Percutaneous • Zadek's osteotomy • Classification • Calcaneoplasty
- Management

KEY POINTS

- Surgical treatment of posterior heel pain and Achilles insertional tendinopathy and understanding of the pathophysiology of the condition have improved.
- The treatment modalities have changed because of technological advances, including endoscopy and minimally invasive surgery, and fixation of tendon onto bone with suture anchors.
- Modern techniques allow earlier functional recovery, lesser insult to tissues through smaller portals, be it minimally invasive surgery or endoscopic management.

HAGLUND'S DEFORMITY HISTORICAL PERSPECTIVE

Swedish orthopedic surgeon Patrick Haglund, who gave his name to the condition in 1928, believed more 'cultured people' developed this condition, because they wore either high heels or stiff-soled shoes while playing golf or hockey.[1] However, this conditions was described even before that by 2 physicians, one of whom was in Vienna and give his name to it as Albert's disease in 1893.[2,3]

The authors have nothing to disclose.
Cardiff Regional Foot & Ankle Surgery Unit, Department of Trauma & Orthopaedic Surgery, University Hospital Llandough & University Hospital Wales, Cardiff & Vale University Health Board, Penlan Road, Llandough, Wales, CF64 2XX, UK
* Corresponding author. Well Field, South Road, Sully, Penarth, Cardiff, Wales CF62 5TY, UK.
E-mail address: turab.syed@gmail.com

Foot Ankle Clin N Am 21 (2016) 641–664
http://dx.doi.org/10.1016/j.fcl.2016.04.004
1083-7515/16/$ – see front matter © 2016 Elsevier Inc. All rights reserved.

It has been associated with various types of shoes as reflected by various names like pump bumps,[4] high heel,[5] and winter heel.[6] Some other names used for this are calcaneus altus, cucumber heel, high prow heel,[5] and hatchet-shaped heel.[7] It must be distinguished from Haglund's disease, which refers to osteonecrosis of the accessory navicular.[8]

The term Halgund's deformity refers to an enlargement of the posterior superior/lateral calcaneum (**Fig. 1**). This can cause impingement of the retrocalcaneal bursa and Achilles insertion, and results in irritation of these and other structures such as the superficial bursa, the bone itself, and the enthesis organ made of the cartilaginous surfaces of the posterior calcaneum and Achilles tendon as well. This symptomatic irritation is referred to as Haglund's syndrome and includes Achilles insertional tendonopathy.

Clinical Features

The patient with symptomatic Haglund's syndrome has a painful, red, irritated heel with a palpable and visible osseous prominence on the lateral aspect of the postero-superior heel. This is often associated with Achilles insertional tendinopathy, retrocalcaneal bursitis, and superficial adventitious Achilles tendon bursitis.[9] The patient complains of enlargement of the posterior heel and difficulty with footwear and sport. The posterolateral surface can become very enlarged and reddened.

ETIOLOGY

Bursitis of the retrocalcaneal space is often of idiopathic origin.[10,11] However, this is an attrition injury and therefore training—and especially running—is a risk factor. With the increasing popularity of running, there has been an increase in the incidence.[12,13] However, it is not confined to athletes, in 1 series of 58 patients, nearly one-third did not participate in vigorous physical activity.[14]

Myerson and McGarvey[15] have noted that a tight gastrocnemius complex, hyper-pronation, cavus foot, and obesity[16–19] can predispose to degeneration, attrition, mechanical abrasion, and chemical irritation that leads to a chronic inflammatory response to the heel. Other authors, too, have described that the patient has a high arched cavus foot with particular narrow heel. However, a recent paper by Shibuya and colleagues[20] found no clinically significant difference in calcaneal inclination between those with or without insertional Achilles tendinosis.

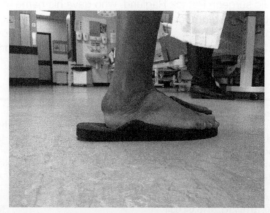

Fig. 1. Showing Haglund's deformity on the posterolateral aspect of the heel.

A cross-sectional study by Kraemer and colleagues[21] in 2012 involving elite and recreational athletes identified a positive family history as a significant solitary risk factor for Achilles tendinopathy, increasing the risk by 5-fold. Some authors advise laboratory tests to exclude conditions like diabetes,[22,23] gout, or rheumatoid arthritis[24] seronegative spondyloarthropathies (Reiter's syndrome, ankylosing spondylitis),[25–27] all of which can affect the enthesis organ.

Earlier studies showed tendinopathy to be more prevalent among older people,[28,29] possibly because there is accumulation of the effect over time[30] and age-related changes in tendon structure and biomechanics result in decreased loading capacity and regenerative capacity of the tendons.[31] Male gender is considered to be a risk factor for Achilles tendinopathy.[32] However, in track and field athletes over 40 years of age, Longo and colleagues[33] did not find a difference in risk between men and women.

Anatomy and Biomechanics

Anatomy of the achilles enthesis and retrocalcaneal bursa

The Achilles tendon is the largest in the body. It has a distal insertion of approximately 1×2 cm and inserts approximately 2 cm distal to posterosuperior edge of the calcaneal tuberosity. The posterior aspect of the calcaneum can be divided into 3 anatomic subsegments,[34] the inferior third is continuous with the plantar aspect of the calcaneum where the fibers of the plantar aponeurosis and fibers from Achilles tendon are attached. The central one-third of the calcaneum is trapezoidal in shape and has multiple grooves and ridges and is the site of attachment of the Achilles tendon.

It was previously thought that the Achilles inserted at the border between middle and inferior posterior calcaneal facets.[35–37] However, Ballal and coworkers[38] in 2014 showed that both the middle and inferior facets are areas of attachment of the tendon. The middle facet has the soleus attachment medially and laterally the lateral head of gastrocnemius. The inferior facet has the attachment of the medial head of gastrocnemius.

The insertions extend medially and laterally, anastomosing with the deep fascia in the form of a crescent.[39] The superior one-third of the calcaneum is triangular shaped with its apex superiorly. The retrocalcaneal bursa is present at this surface.

The Achilles tendon is the culmination of the triceps surae complex, made of muscles and tendons of gastrocnemius, soleus, and plantaris, controlling plantar motion at ankle and subtalar joint across which it inserts and, to an extent, knee flexion owing to the origin of the gastrocnemius from behind the femoral condyles. There is a complex rotatory arrangement of fibers in the tendon where they spiral approximately 90°, with the medial fibers rotating posteriorly and the posterior fibers rotating laterally as they insert onto calcaneum.[40] Plantaris involvement can be difficult to diagnose, because it is known to have a variable insertion patterns along the anteromedial Achilles.

Two bursae are associated with the Achilles tendon, the subcutaneous bursa, known as the Achilles tendon bursa or adventitial bursa between the skin and the tendon and the retrocalcaneal bursa between the Achilles tendon and the calcaneum and sits on top of the posterosuperior aspect of calcaneum (see **Fig. 1**). Both can become inflamed in Haglund's syndrome.

The retrocalcaneal bursa has a volume of 1 to 1.5 mL and is horse shoe shaped. The average length of the bursal legs is 22 mm with a width of each leg of 4 mm. The width of the bursal body is 8 mm. The retrocalcaneal bursa has an anterior bursal wall composed of fibrocartilage laid over the calcaneum, and the posterior wall is indistinguishable from the thin epitenon of the Achilles tendon. This disc shaped structure lies over the posterosuperior aspect of calcaneus and has a concave aspect anteriorly.

Recently, it has been found that the bursa could be unicameral (single cavity) or bicameral (made up of a smaller medially based cavity and larger laterally based cavity).[38] This maintains a constant distance between the axis of ankle joint and the insertion of the Achilles tendon.

If the posterior prominence is not present, there is a shortening of the distance between the ankle joint and the insertion of the Achilles tendon during the dorsiflexion. As this lever arm is shortened, there is a consequential effect on the ability of the gastrocnemius and soleus complex. This projection in fact works as a 'cam,' pushing the Achilles tendon posteriorly as the foot dorsiflexes and vice versa, allowing the tension of gastrocnemius–soleus muscle group through the Achilles tendon to remain constant with dorsiflexion and plantar flexion as happens in metacarpophalangeal joint of hand.[41] The bursa lies in front of the Achilles tendon between it and the posterior calcaneus and is bound at the front by a fat pad, which appears as Kaeger's fat pad on radiographs. In plain lateral ankle radiographs, disruption of this fat pad is diagnostic of retrocalcaneal bursitis.

The insertional region of the Achilles was well studied by Rufai and colleagues[42] in 1995 who showed the tendency for cartilagelike changes to develop within the tendon on the stress-shielded side of the enthesis, leading to intratendinous bone formation through endochondral ossification. Benjamin and colleagues[43] showed that calcification and spur formation at the insertion does not depend on inflammation or prior microtears. These develop to increase the surface area at the bone–tendon interface to protect the area from increased mechanical load. This process can be described on the same rationale as osteophytes developing to increase the surface area in an arthritic joint.

The vascular supply for the posterior heel forms an arterial network composed of the calcaneal anastomotic vessels from posterior tibial artery, peroneal artery, medial and lateral calcaneal arteries, and further branches from the lateral and medial plantar arteries. Because these vessels are developed in childhood, they supply the calcaneal apophysis and the insertion of the Achilles tendon along with the plantaris and other surrounding structures. Although there is a 'water shed' region about 2 to 6 cm proximal to insertion as described by Lagergren and Lindholm[44] in 1958. In contrast, the vascularity of the enthesis region is excellent though it does show a decrease in relation to age as shown by Astrom and Westlin[45] in 1994.

Biomechanics of achilles enthesis

Tendons not only transmit forces generated from muscles to bone, but also act as a buffer to absorb external forces to prevent or reduce damage to the muscles.[46] Loading of the Achilles tendon reaches up to 9 kN during running (corresponding with 12.5 times the body weight), 2.6 kN during slow walking, and less than 1 kN during cycling.[47]

The posterior fibers of the Achilles tendon sustain more force owing to an increased lever arm, which results in more dystrophy of these fibers.[34] This dystrophy results in degeneration of the tendon and deposition of calcification at the superficial fibers, creating pain in the insertional region of calcaneum. Biomechanical studies have shown that dorsiflexion of foot increases pressure on the retrocalcaneal bursa and, conversely, pressure is reduced by plantarflexion of the foot.[48,49] The main function of the bursa is to act as a spacer between the axes of the ankle joint and the Achilles tendon.

It has been noted[50,51] that calcification of the Achilles and posterior calcaneal spurs were 8 ($P = .004$) and 9.2 ($P < .001$) times higher in patients with posterior heel pain than those who were pain free. Sella and colleagues[8] have postulated that a posterior calcaneal step effectively increases the length of calcaneum, which in turn increases tension on the Achilles tendon. It is thought that calcification in Achilles tendon results from prominent bursal projection, which tents the Achilles and hence results in degenerative tendons.

As the Achilles inserts into the calcaneum, subtalar motion can subject the tendon fibers to an uneven rotational force, which can lead to an imbalance at the insertion of the tendon. This is particularly noticeable in runners whose feet hyperpronate during midstance causing internal rotational forces on tibia. Later as the knee is extended, this now causes opposite (external) rotation force on the tibia. These contradictory forces impart high stresses on the insertion of the Achilles.[52]

Root and colleagues[53] in 1977 debated the biomechanics of patients with Haglund's deformity. They thought that abnormal subtalar joint motion led to development of retrocalcaneal bursitis. This is because the subtalar joint would try to compensate for either a fixed rear foot varus or a rigid forefoot valgus. The position in a rear foot varus would make the posterosuperior corner more prominent and compensatory pronation of foot would cause sheer forces at heel. Similarly, in the rigid forefoot valgus, supination at subtalar joint will cause inversion of heel and increase in calcaneal inclination angle. Before this, Sgarlato first described abnormal pronation in the foot as a precursor to symptoms[54] and later effect of lengthening Achilles on foot mechanics.[55]

ASSESSMENT AND INVESTIGATION

The diagnosis of Haglund's syndrome is generally straightforward with obvious posterior heel pain, swelling, and redness. Tenderness is felt posterior, but it is very important to discern the precise distribution of the tenderness because this is very helpful for surgical planning. If there is rubbing and pain on the posterior heel, then this needs to be reduced by removing or rotating the bone. If the distal Achilles is tender, then this is likely to be diseased and is likely to need addressing with either debridement or flexor hallucis longus tendon transfer. If the pain is anterior to the Achilles either in the fat pad, retrocalcaneal burse or posterior superior prominence of the calcaneum, then decompression alone may be sufficient.

Plain film radiographs are not necessary for diagnosis; however, the presence of bony spurs in the tendon makes one more concerned about the state of the Achilles tendon. The presence of a large number of bone or spurs elsewhere can suggest ankylosing spondylitis. A posterior Achilles spur may be a negative prognostic factor for endoscopy on its own.

Assessment for gastrocnemius contracture is important.

Plain radiographs are helpful in planning a Zadek osteotomy to assess the calcaneal pitch angle and plan the osteotomy. However, they are not helpful in determining the size of the deformity or amount of bone removal, although a number of measures have been proposed.[5,49,50,56–63]

MRI scan is the investigation of choice for surgical planning, because this gives a much better understanding of the structures that are affected in Haglund's syndrome (**Fig. 2**). If the tendon is very diseased, then an aggressive surgical approach is necessary either as a debridement and reattachment or, if severe, then a flexor hallucis longus transfer may even be required. The best results for endoscopy in the senior author's experience are the presence of retrocalcaneal bursitis with superior bone edema and no or mild Achilles tendonopathy.

CONSERVATIVE MANAGEMENT OF HAGLUND'S SYNDROME

A detailed review of conservative management is not within the remit of this article. However, although conservative treatment in the form of rest, activity modification,

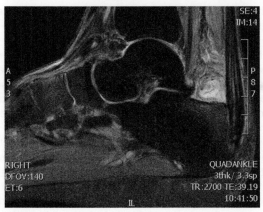

Fig. 2. MRI showing the retrocalcaneal bursitis, with changes in the Achilles and superior calcaneum.

footwear modification, ice, and analgesia are very important, the success rate of shockwave therapy and gastrocnemius stretching are less than for midsubstance Achilles tendonopathy. Furthermore, these treatments may be uncomfortable.

Open Surgical Management

Open haglund deformity debridement
Superoposterior calcaneal resection has been described to be carried out from a posterolateral, posteromedial, or a dual incision, and even using a Cincinnati incision.[64] This is reserved for situations using just debridement of the retrocalcaneal bursa and posterior superior corner of the calcaneum and is the open equivalent of the endoscopic approach.

The results of open surgery have generally shown good results.[12,65] However the postoperative protocols generally require long periods of immobilization[12,66,67] and recovery can take a long time. Furthermore, immobilization carries the subsequent risk of new adhesions and scar tissue formation because functional rehabilitation cannot start immediately. Hence, this leads to delayed complications such as stiffness and pain.

However, although these studies have mainly occurred in a young population recovery has not been uniform and as Angermann[68] showed in 40 patients (40 heels) for the same indications using a posterolateral incision and allowing immediate weight bearing in 37 patients. Complications were 1 superficial heel infection, 1 hematoma, and 2 delayed skin healing. At an average follow-up of 6 years, 50% of the patients were cured, 20% were improved, 20% were unchanged, and 10% were worse.

Other studies, too, have shown failure rates of up to 25% to 30%, and reoperation.[69,70] Huber and Waldis[71] found a considerable amount of residual complaints in 32 patients who were clinically and radiologically reviewed at a mean follow-up of 18.6 years after being treated for Haglund's resection. Out of 32 patients, 14 had soft tissue problems, not enough resection in 8 patients, and 2 patients had new bone formation.

Open surgery requires extensive exposure and it can be difficult to be sure of the exact amount of bone resected on the medial side unless a double approach with an additional medial incision is used.

With open surgery, various other complications have been reported, like weakness of the calcaneus after removing the posterosuperior bony prominence,[72] persistent pain,[73] and hypoesthesia in the area of the scar.[65]

Open achilles detachment, debridement, and reattachment

Other authors have used a more aggressive approach using a midline incision to overcome the difficulties of visualization from a medial or lateral approach from complete detachment of the Achilles tendon. A biomechanical study from Kolodziej and colleagues[74] suggested that 50% of the tendon attachment can be safely debrided with minimal risk of rerupture. However, Nunley and colleagues[75] technique debrided up to 70% of insertion of Achilles tendon using a central incision and without augmenting it, and were able to achieve 96% satisfaction with good function at 7 years.

Reattachment has been described by using various materials ranging from using simple bone anchors,[76] screws, or transosseous sutures in single or double row fashion.[77] Where a proper reattachment is performed the tendon maintains normal plantarflexion.[78,79] Although biomechanically single-row or double-row repairs result in similar peak loads to failure,[80] but in complete detachments the footprint of the insertion may be better restored if double-row techniques are used.

Calder and Saxby[81] in their review of 52 patients noted that failures were uncommon and that central tendon splitting approach to be safer. The results have generally been good[82] in terms of pain relief and function.

The major concerns with this procedure are the prolonged period of immobilization and non-weight bearing, the soft tissue complications and prolonged recovery. With a double-row technique, weight bearing can commence earlier[83] but in this series 2 patients (5%) had wound healing problems with 7% of the total series requiring further surgery because of this. In another series by Brunner and associates,[84] complications were low but time to recovery was such that they recommended studies should not assess patients at less than 1 year and that 2-year follow-up was the minimum. Six of their 36 patients would not recommend the surgery because of this, although the overall success rate was 86%.

Open flexor hallucis longus tendon transfer

Flexor hallucis longus tendon transfer is rarely indicated in Haglund's syndrome, unless the tendon is very diseased. However, even then there is little evidence that it adds any advantage over debridement and reattachment alone.[85,86]

Minimal Access Surgery

Endoscopic calcaneoplasty

Eda van Dyk first performed endoscopic resection of the posterosuperior calcaneus during a fellowship with Dr Lanny Johnson in 1991. Later he, along with Van Djik from Amsterdam, carried out this procedure in a consecutive patient series in which 20 patients were included and gave this technique the name of "endoscopic calcaneoplasty." Since then, various techniques and portals have been described.[87]

In van Dijk and colleagues'[88] initial series of 20 patients, 19 had good to excellent results with return to sport after 12 weeks. Jerosch and colleagues[89] from Neuss, Germany, in their first publication studied 81 patients for an average of 35.3 months after endoscopic calcaneoplasty. The Ogilvie-Harris score was excellent in 41 patients, good in 34, fair in 3, and poor in 3. The patients with poor results were revised with an open approach and these patients had ossification of the Achilles tendon. In his subsequent series[90] of 164 patients (ages 16–64 years) from 1999 to 2010 with an average follow-up of 46.3 months (range, 8–120), he showed that 71 patients had good results and 84 patients had excellent results according to the

Ogilvie-Harris score. Only 5 patients showed fair results and 4 patients reported poor results. In 61 patients, preoperative MRI showed a partial rupture of the Achilles tendon close to the insertion site. There were no cases of a complete tear at the time of follow-up. Only minor postoperative complications were observed. Their experience showed good and excellent results in more than 90% of patients.

Ortmann and McBryd[91] reported on 28 patients (30 heels) with an average follow-up of 35 months, similar to Jerosch's first study.[90] The American Orthopaedic Foot & Ankle Society score improved from 62 preoperatively to[92] postoperatively. There were 26 excellent results, 3 good results, and 1 poor result. No wound complications or postoperative infections were noted, but 2 patients required open surgery at 3 weeks because they sustained Achilles tendon rupture.

Jerosch[90] has described the minimally invasive endoscopic calcaneoplasty as a suitable alternative to the open technique for symptomatic Haglund's syndrome. This can achieve reproducible results, allows an excellent differentiation of different disorders, and has fewer complications than the open technique with short learning curve.

Complete avulsion after endoscopic calcaneoplasty has not been reported. Although Achilles tendon avulsions after open resection of a Haglund spur have been described in the literature. The reason for this may be that, with endoscopic calcaneoplasty, the surgeon protects the medial and lateral insertional fibers of the Achilles, which protect the tendon, whereas during the open resection these fibers also are released.[91]

Irritation of the whole heel has been described as a possible complication in early endoscopic calcaneoplasty series.[73]

The clinical negative predictor for open calcaneoplasty is older age, association with intratendinous injury, and the extent of the resection.[93] Open calcaneoplasty has complications related to delayed wound healing, edema, painful scar, and hypothesia.[65,94,95] A multicenter retrospective series of open and endoscopic techniques by Bohu and colleagues[94] in 2009 proposed endoscopic techniques for main body tendinopathies and retrocalcaneal pathologies.

Surgical treatment of Achilles Insertional by debridement of enesthesis using endoscopic techniques has shown good results.[96,97] Systematic reviews of open versus endoscopic debridement have shown better results with the endoscopic approach.[92] Postoperatively, patients are managed in a boot, commencing early weight-bearing and motion, with a faster recovery and better results than with an open debridement.

Zadek's calcaneal osteotomy

Following Haglund's treatment methodology of only resecting the prominent postero-superior calcaneum, Zadek[98] in 1939 in his seminal paper described his procedure where he carried out a rotational osteotomy of the posterior calcaneum in young female patients with uniformly good results. He managed them using only catgut suture through the bone to hold it together and a cast in equinus for 5 weeks while allowing them to bear weight after a couple of weeks by using a felt under the heel of plaster of Paris cast. He compared this with the treatment of hallux, where one would not just remove the burse and consider the procedure satisfactory; yet this is often done in Achilles bursitis without attacking the underlying bony abnormality. He described the object of the operation as the removal of the underlying bony prominence and incidentally the excision of the chronically inflamed bursa. He used a transverse incision as well as a longitudinal one, but found the longitudinal approach to be more satisfactory. He removed a wedge from the os calcis at a point of one-half to three-quarters of an inch from its posterior border and base of the wedge was one-quarter inch wide with the apex of the wedge present toward the sole. The posterior fragment of bone was countersunk by means of boneset and mallet and approximation maintained by a couple of chromic catgut sutures. He described his series of 3 female patients, two were 22 and one was 21 years old.

The mechanism of action of the Zadek osteotomy is likely to be mulitmodal, but may in part be owing to a reduction in this lever arm and also an increase in the blood supply to the region by way of an osteotomy, similar to distal radial osteotomies, which increase blood flow to the lunate in wrist for Keinbock's disease. In addition, it may alter the mechanics of the Achilles tendon and decompress the enthesis.

Following on from him, Keck and Kelly[99] described the procedure in a much bigger group (18 patients compared with only 3 from Zadek's series). They showed a good outcome in 18 patients with 26 symptomatic heels. Of these heels, 5 were treated with a dorsally based wedge osteotomy of the calcaneus (which later was called a Keck and Kelly osteotomy) to decrease the prominence of the posterosuperior corner of the heel. The posterior fragment was simply impacted into the anterior fragment in 4 heels; in 1 heel, a staple was used for fixation. Out of these 5 repairs, 3 were rated as good or fair results and 2 rated as poor results, although they themselves concluded that there were too few osteotomies performed to properly evaluate this procedure.

However, it is to be noted that for the intervening 25 years or so from 1939 article of Zadek[99] to that of Keck and Kelly 1965 in the *Journal of Bone and Joint Surgery*, there were no publications on the Zadek osteotomy. Keck and Kelly limited its indications to patients with a strong calcaneal angle of inclination. Miller and Vogel[100] in 1989 performed the osteotomy along with smoothing of the posterosuperior process of the calcaneum and also performed internal osteosynthesis.

The position of the closing wedge osteotomy is critical; if it is placed too far anterior or posterior, it can affect the subtalar joint or Achilles insertion (**Figs. 3** and **5–7**). Another problem is occurrence of sharp posteroinferior bony prominence requiring further surgery as the heel pad shifts posteriorly and superiorly. It also changes the shape of the posterior aspect of the heel and some authors find that this makes the heel slightly wider though the posterior eminence is reduced. Myerson and McGarvey[15] have advised against osteotomy routinely because of increased morbidity compared with a simpler lateral resection except in those with deformed heels.

In 1995, a modification of the Keck and Kelly was described by Dennis Martin[101] (**Fig. 4**), which allowed anterior advancement of the posterior calcaneus and Achilles tendon without increasing tension on the plantar soft tissues. Keck and Kelly

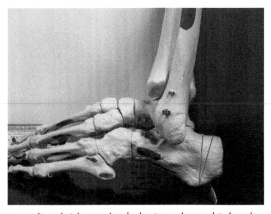

Fig. 3. The osteotomy exit point is proximal plantar calcaneal tubercle.

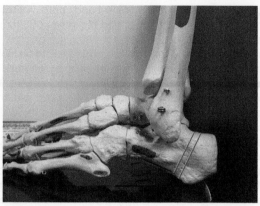

Fig. 4. Modified Keck and Kelly osteotomy. The osteotomy removes a rectangular piece (4–6 mm wide) and both osteotomy points are distal to the plantar calcaneal tubercle.

described a wedge-type osteotomy along the posterior body of the calcaneus to relocate the posterior insertion area and the Achilles tendon to a more anterior and superior position as shown in **Fig. 8**. Concerned by the potential elongation and posterior displacement of the plantar structures including the calcaneal tubercle, the alternative osteotomy design was described as shown in **Fig. 4**. The 5 year retrospective results review of 38 osteotomies on 33 patients showed generally excellent results with low complications and only 3 patents with ongoing symptoms and only 4 delayed union that eventually healed uneventfully by 6 months.[102] Sural nerve involvement was the most commonly encountered complication. This was seen in 4 patients (12%), 3 of whom went on to require sural nerve resection. After this undesirable complication, the authors changed their incision from a diagonal one to a longitudinal one across the long axis of calcaneum (see **Figs. 3** and **4**).

Zadek's osteotomy controls the position of tuberosity in sagittal plane. It is a dorsal closing wedge that allows the posterior and superior angle of the tuberosity to be brought forward, reducing the conflict with the anterior face of the Achilles tendon. The position of vertex of osteotomy is of paramount importance, because this determines whether or not the heel is placed horizontally. If the vertex is kept posterior, a

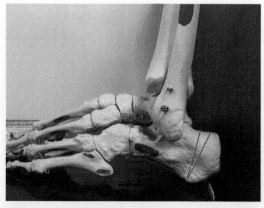

Fig. 5. Zadek's osteotomy with a posterior vertex.

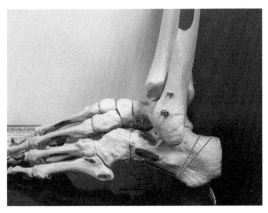

Fig. 6. Vertex anterior of osteotomy.

forward rotation of the tuberosity is obtained (see **Fig. 3**; **Fig. 5**). However, if the vertex is anterior as in **Fig. 6**, an elevation of the tuberosity is achieved resulting in horizontalization of the heel in a cavus foot preoperatively (**Figs. 6** and **7**).

There is a lack of literature on Zadek's osteotomy in the English language literature; it is more commonly performed in France as an alternative to simple exostectomy.[103] The Chauveaux–Liet angle is represented by the difference between the angle of verticalization (α) and morphologic angle (β) of the calcaneus (Chauveaux–Liet angle = $\alpha - \beta$; **Fig. 9**). Angle α is the calcaneal pitch angle or angle of verticalization of calcaneus, described as the intersection of the baseline tangent to the anterior tubercle and the medial tuberosity with the horizontal surface. The angle β is formed between the vertical line tangent to the most posterior point of greater tuberosity and the straight line joining this point to the apex of the posterosuperior crest. A Chauveaux–Liet angle of more than 12° is considered abnormal in conditions like Haglund's deformity (see **Figs. 9** and **10**).

With the algorithm of Chauveaux and Liet, an angle greater than 30° is a good indication for primary Zadek's osteotomy.[90] Each degree of wedge elevates the tuberosity by same degrees as shown in **Figs. 6** and **8**. If further superior migration is required,

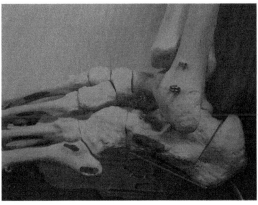

Fig. 7. Effect of reducing calcaneal pitch angle and horizontalization the heel in a vertex anterior osteotomy.

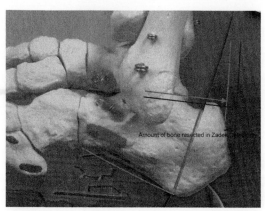

Fig. 8. Effect of elevating the tuberosity. Blue arrow before and red after Zadek's osteotomy.

the inferior cortex can be cut to allow to do that (see **Fig. 8**). This makes osteotomy potentially unstable and requires 2 screws to control rotation as well (see **Fig. 8**).

Calcaneal osteotomy can be carried out both by minimally invasive surgery and open techniques. The advantage of the open technique is that it is a quicker procedure, although it is a large wound that takes time to heal and is in an area where blood supply is poor. The advantage of minimally invasive surgery is that it can be performed through a small incision, which heals very well. However, this technique does increase the operating time because radiology is used to position K wires and then the osteotomy is made using a high torque but low speed special Shannon and wedge burr using a pencil driver under fluoroscopic guidance (**Figs. 11–13**).

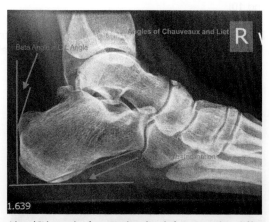

Fig. 9. Chauveaux–Liet (CL) angle for Haglund's deformity: the difference between the angle of verticalization (α) and morphologic angle (β) of the calcaneus (CL angle = $\alpha - \beta$). Angle α is the calcaneal pitch angle or angle of verticalization of calcaneus described as the intersection of the baseline tangent to the anterior tubercle and the medial tuberosity with the horizontal surface. The angle β is formed between the vertical line tangent to the most posterior point of greater tuberosity and the straight line joining this point to the apex of the posterosuperior crest.

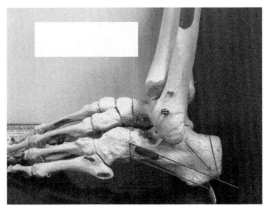

Fig. 10. The "new angle" and the amount of bone to be resected. 1, Inclination line; 2, base of flare of the anterior calcaneal process; 3, line parallel to inclination; 4, base of flare of superior calcaneal tuberosity; 5, new angle; and 6, bone to be removed.

OPERATIVE TECHNIQUES
Surgical Decision Making

The senior authors' management plan is shown in **Table 1**. This plan primarily is based on 4 parameters: the state of the tendon, the site of pain, the size of the bony prominence, and the calcaneal pitch angle. Ideally, one would just use an endoscopic approach, because it has minimal morbidity and excellent results with the quickest recovery. However, it has been shown the presence of a spur within the tendon has a negative effect on outcome, as discussed. In our experience, however, this is less important than the state of tendon and the functional ability of the patient, because this can be done supine with immediate weight-bearing and a quicker recovery. However, if the posterior heel is tender and not just anterior to the Achilles in the fat pad, bursa, or posterosuperior prominence, then endoscopy alone will not be sufficient.

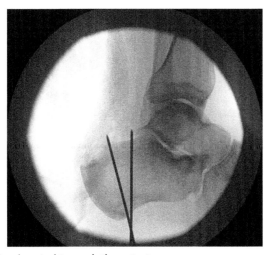

Fig. 11. Two K wires inserted to mark the osteotomy.

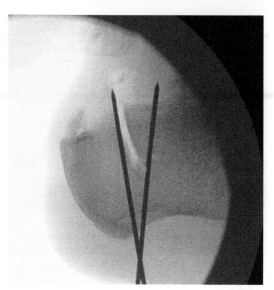

Fig. 12. Osteotomy being guided by K wires.

A modest posterior bony protrusion can rotate around with a Zadek's osteotomy, but a very severe one will not correct fully. Although again it may be preferable to perform this to an open procedure in patients who can only undergo supine surgery with immediate/early weight-bearing.

In patients with an elevated calcaneal pitch angle, it is helpful to reduce this angle by performing a Zadek's osteotomy with the apex anterior to the plantar calcaneal tuberosity (**Fig. 6**). In those with a normal or low angle, this angle must be preserved and it is preferable to make apex at the plantar tubercle or even posterior to it (**Fig. 5**).

If the posterior bony deformity is very large, then an open calcaneoplasty is required particularly if the tendon is very diseased. The presence of medial pain also points to an open approach. If the tendon is very diseased, then a flexor hallucis longus tendon transfer can be performed endoscopically, although this is required infrequently.

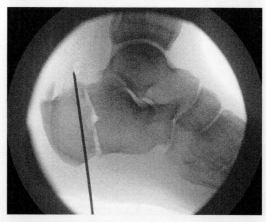

Fig. 13. Zadek osteotomy completed.

Table 1
The senior author's management protocol for Haglund's syndrome

Stage	Achilles Tendon	Ossification	Posterior Bony Prominence	Management
1	Normal/mild isolated bone island	No spur or <7 mm	Minimal protrusion (<5 mm)	Endoscopic calcaneoplasty and bursal excision
2a	Moderate tendon	Spur 7–15 mm	Tender posterior heel Protrusion <10 mm	Minimally invasive Zadek's osteotomy
2b	Moderate tendon Marked enthesitis	Spur 7–15 mm	Tender posterior heel Protrusion 10–15 mm	Minimally invasive Zadek's osteotomy plus Endoscopic calcaneoplasty
3	Severe	—	Medial bony pain Protrusion >12 mm	Open calcaneoplasty With or without flexor hallucis longus tendon transfer

Endoscopic calcaneoplasty technique

This technique has been well-described in a previous paper[90] and is not addressed in detail here. The author's preference is for a supine approach with the leg internally rotated to allow good access to the lateral part of the calcaneus. This is always large than the medial portion and is also where the bone edema almost always commences and is, therefore, at its worst (**Fig. 14**).

A 4-mm scope is used with a 4.5-mm hooded shaver (**Fig. 15**) for the soft tissue and bone removal. This is continued until there is no gap between tendon and bone (see **Fig. 10**; **Fig. 16**). Pay particular attention to the medial and lateral corners because there is a tendency to undercut these areas. Assess for any impingement in full dorsiflexion of the foot (see **Figs. 15** and **16**).

Intraoperative image intensifier is used to confirm adequate removal of bone. If there is a step in the bone that may cause sharp rubbing on footwear, then this can be removed. A beaver blade in introduced and used to release the tendon off the bone gradually. A small amount of elevation does not require reattachment. However, if this is significant then suture anchors can be passed percutaneously through the

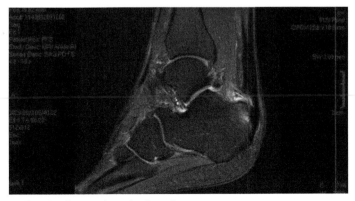

Fig. 14. MRI showing bone edema in the calcaneum.

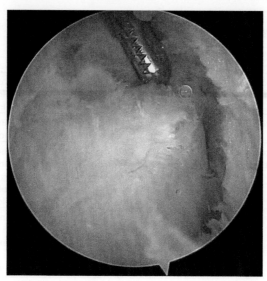

Fig. 15. Endoscopic image showing Haglund's deformity and Achilles insertion.

tendon and the skin open superficially to allow these to be tied off. Or these can be tied off internally by pulling the sutures through into the retrocalcaneal space and out of the instrument portal and tied off under direct vision with a knot pusher.

Minimally invasive Zadek's osteotomy

Patient positioning and setup It is preferable to have the patient supine, because this position allows for concomitant endoscopy and many of the nonathletic patients will be overweight. A bolster is placed under the patient's thigh to elevate the foot and sandbag under the ipsilateral buttock to ensure that the foot points directly up. This position enables a true lateral view on fluoroscopy that comes from the same side

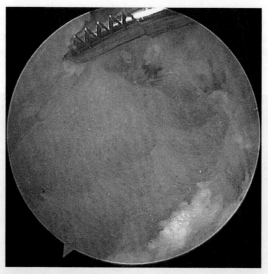

Fig. 16. Showing endoscopic calcaneoplasty performed. The posterior ridge (just next to the shaver) must be shaved.

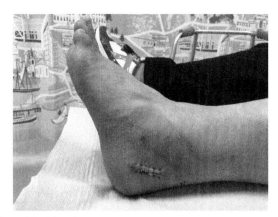

Fig. 17. A 2-cm lateral incision for percutaneous osteotomy.

and is set up over the top of the patient. The most important reason, however, is that this positioning enables the surgeon to visualize the heel and ensure that the burr is perpendicular to the heel at all times.

Surgical approach This is not a truly percutaneous approach, because the osteotomy can be quite long and therefore it is the senior authors preference to make a lateral skin incision of 2 cm to allow for some translation of the burr (**Fig. 17**). The incision is marked out with fluoroscopy based on the wedge required. If the pitch angle is increased, the apex will be anterior to the plantar tuberosity. If it is normal or reduced, then the apex is at the tuberosity or even further posterior. However, this reduces the amount of rotation and thus posterior pump bump correction. The skin is incised and then blunt dissection is performed to expose the calcaneum. The peroneal tendons are superior and the osteotomy should be in the internervous plane (see **Fig. 17**).

Surgical procedure A 3 × 20-mm Shannon burr is used for the initial osteotomy and then either a 3.1-mm or 4.1-mm wedge burr for the bone removal. Saline is run onto the burr to cool it down, but this will not completely control the heat. Thus, the burr must be removed regularly to clean the debris because this buildup increases heat generation and it also allows the burr to cool. The high-torque, low-speed burr is set at a maximum of 300 rpm at a gear ratio of 20:1.

To guide the osteotomy in the early experience, two 2-mm guidewires can be inserted from inferior to mark the boundaries of the osteotomy (**Fig. 11**). Be careful

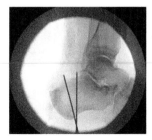
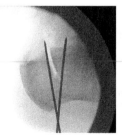
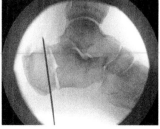

Fig. 18. Using K wires as a jig. Initially, 2 K wires are used and are inserted under fluoroscopic control from sole of foot. These effectively act as a jig and stop Shannon Burr from slipping away from the triangular area/wedge, which is burred away.

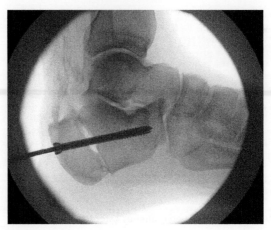

Fig. 19. Zadek osteotomy with screw in situ.

not to damage these; the burr is very sharp. Start by marking out the osteotomy on the lateral cortex and then using this as a guide to the medial cortex. Use the note of the burr and the resistance of the burr to guide the depth.

Bone removal is performed and can take some time (**Figs. 12, 13,** and **18**). Care must be taken not to go too close to the posterior subtalar joint. The plantar cortex should be preserved (**Figs. 19** and **20**). Regularly test the osteotomy to see if it can

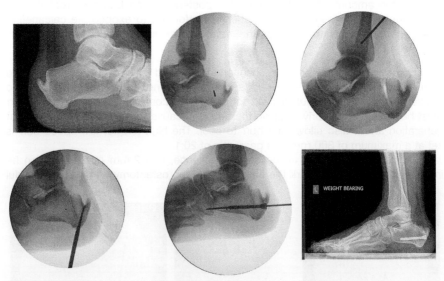

Fig. 20. Preoperative and postoperative radiographs. No retrocalcaneal bursitis is present. The pain was posterior over the spur. The patient had multiple comorbidities, including diabetes and respiratory disease, that prevented him from having prone surgery. Therefore, supine isolated Zadek osteotomy was performed. However, this approach was modified because he had a normal calcaneal pitch angle. The apex of the osteotomy was posterior to the plantar tubercle to prevent flattening of the foot. This reduces the amount of rotation possible, but can still be sufficient.

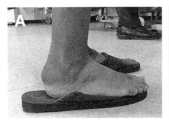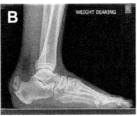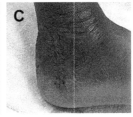

Fig. 21. (*A*) Preoperative image shows a large posterior bony eminence this was the site of pain rather than the degeneration within the Achilles tendon. (*B*) Preoperative radiograph. (*C*) At 4 weeks after the operation. Patient commenced weight bearing in boot and range of motion exercises at 2 weeks.

close. This does not need to be full as the screw insertion will complete the closure. Once adequate bone has been removed then a 6.5-mm screw can be inserted from posterior and the head buried (**Figs. 11–13; 18–20**).

Postoperative management Ideally, the patient is placed in a plaster back-slab for 2 weeks with no weight bearing to allow the soft tissues to settle. However, in larger patients or those unable to not bear weight, it is stable enough to permit weight bearing with crutches in a boot. Thromboprophylaxis is used.

At 2 weeks, the cast is removed and the patient is placed into a boot. This can be removed for bed and gentle range of motion exercises. However, it must be on for all weight bearing, which can now commence, using 2 crutches for 4 weeks **Fig. 21**.

At 6 weeks, radiographs are taken and the patient can start passive range of motion exercises and increase weight bearing to be free of crutches. Usually, the patient can go into a sneaker after a further 2 to 4 weeks and full rehabilitation can commence. This can be progressed through depending on pain (see **Fig. 21**).

Complications Nerve injury is very uncommon; if it does occur, it affects the lateral nerves. Sometimes if the patient is large and weight bearing is commenced early, the heel can swell and be slow to settle.

SUMMARY

Surgical treatment of posterior heel pain and Achilles insertional tendinopathy has improved over last century as has our understanding of the pathophysiology of the condition. The treatment modalities have changed because of technological advances, whether it be use of endoscopy or minimally invasive surgery or fixation technique of tendon onto bone with suture anchors.

From the original days of Zadek, where catgut was used for osteosynthesis, we now have percutaneous screws with reliable and stable fixation. Modern techniques allow earlier functional recovery with lesser insult to tissues through smaller portals, be it minimally invasive surgery or endoscopic management of heel conditions. The principle osteotomy is the same, but its execution is different. Our understanding why and how osteotomy helps in these condition has certainly improved, with more understanding of biomechanical mechanism involved!

REFERENCES

1. Haglund P. Beitrag zur uliwik der Achilesse have. Z Orthop Chir 1928;49.
2. Albert E. Achillodynia. Vienna Med J 1893;34:49–58.

3. White CS. Retrocalcaneal bursitis. NY Med J 1893;98:263.
4. Dickinson PH, Coutts MB, Woodward EP, et al. Tendo achillis bursitis. report of twenty-one cases. J Bone Joint Surg Am 1966;48(1):77–81.
5. Fowler A, Philip JF. Abnormalities of the calcaneus as a cause of painful heel: its diagnosis and operative treatment. Br J Surg 1945;32:494–8.
6. Nisbet NW. Tendo achillis bursitis (winter heel). Br Med J 1954;2:1394–5.
7. Dickinson PH, Couts MB, Woodward EP, et al. TendoAchilles bursitis: report of twenty cases. J Bone Joint Surg Am 1966;48A:77–81.
8. Sella EJ, Caminear DS, McLarney EA. Haglund's syndrome. J Foot Ankle Surg 1998;37:110–4.
9. Jerosch J, Nasef NM. Endoscopic calcaneoplasty–rationale, surgical technique, and early results: a preliminary report. Knee Surg Sports Traumatol Arthrosc 2003;11(3):190–5.
10. Schunck J, Jerosch J. Operative treatment of Haglund's syndrome. Basics, indications, procedures, surgical techniques, results and problems. Foot and ankle surgery 2005;11(3):123–30.
11. Ippolito E, Ricciardi-Pollini PT. Invasive retrocalcaneal bursitis: a report on three cases. Foot Ankle 1984;4:204–8.
12. Jones DC, James SL. Partial calcaneal ostectomy for retrocalcaneal bursitis. Am J Sports Med 1984;12(1):72–3.
13. Kvist M. Achilles tendon injuries in athletes. Ann Chir Gynaecol 1991;80(2):188–201.
14. Rolf CMT. Etiology, histopathology, and outcome of surgery in achillodynia. Foot Ankle Int 1997;18:565–9.
15. Myerson MS, McGarvey W. Disorders of the Achilles tendon insertion and Achilles tendinitis. Instr Course Lect 1999;48:211–8.
16. Gaida J, Cook J, Bass S. Adiposity and tendinopathy. Disabil Rehabil 2008;30:1555–62.
17. Scott A, Zwerver J, Grewal N, et al. Lipids, adiposity and tendinopathy: is there a mechanistic link? Critical review. Br J Sports Med 2015;49:984–8.
18. Owens B, Wolf J, Seelig A, et al. Risk factors for lower extremity tendinopathies in military personnel. Orthop J Sports Med 2013;1(1). 2325967113492707.
19. Gaida JE, Alfredson H, Kiss ZS, et al. Asymptomatic Achilles tendon pathology is associated with a central fat distribution in men and aperipheral fat distribution in women: a crosssectional study of 298 individuals. BMC Musculoskelet Disord 2010;2(11):41.
20. Shibuya N, Thorud JC, Agarwal MR, et al. Is calcaneal inclination higher in patients with insertional Achilles tendinosis? A case-controlled, cross-sectional study,. J Foot Ankle Surg 2012;51(6):757–61.
21. Kraemer R, Wuerfel W, Lorenzen J, et al. Analysis of hereditary and medical risk factors in Achilles tendinopathy and Achilles tendon ruptures: a matched pair analysis. Arch Orthop Trauma Surg 2012;132(6):847–53.
22. Irwin TA. Current concepts review: insertional Achilles tendinopathy. Foot Ankle Int 2010;31:933–9.
23. Abate M, Schiavone C, Salini V, et al. Occurrence of tendon pathologies in metabolic disorders. Rheumatology (Oxford) 2013;52:599–608.
24. Hartmann HO. The tendon sheaths and synovial bursae of the foot. Foot Ankle 1981;1:247–96.
25. Kucuksen S, Karahan AY, Erol K. Haglund syndrome with pump bump. Med Arch 2012;66(6):425–7.

26. Gerster JC. Plantar fasciitis and Achilles tendinitis among 150 cases of seronegative spondarthritis. Rheumatol Rehabil 1980;19(4):218–22.
27. Moll JM. Seronegative arthropathies in the foot. Baillieres Clin Rheumatol 1987; 1(2):289–314.
28. Werner RA, Franzblau A, Gell N, et al. A longitudinal study of industrial and clerical workers: predictors of upper extremity tendonitis. J Occup Rehabil 2005;15: 37–46.
29. Maffulli N, Wong J, Almekinders LC. Types and epidemiology of tendinopathy. Clin Sports Med 2003;22:675–92.
30. Rees JD, Maffulli N, Cook J. Management of tendinopathy. Am J Sports Med 2009;37:1855–67.
31. Zhou B, Zhou Y, Tang K. An overview of structure, mechanical properties, and treatment for age-related tendinopathy. J Nutr Health Aging 2014;18:441–8.
32. Van Linschoten R, den Hoed P, de Jongh A. Guideline 'chronic Achilles tendinopathy, in particular tendinosis, in sportsmen/sportswomen'. Ned Tijdschr Geneeskd 2007;151:2319–24.
33. Longo UG, Rittweger J, Garau G, et al. No influence of age, gender, weight, height, and impact profile in Achilles tendinopathy in masters track and field athletes. Am J Sports Med 2009;37:1400–5.
34. Pebbles CF. Evaluation of posterior heel: clinical & radiographic anatomy. Chapter 12. Available at: http://www.podiatryinstitute.com/pdfs/Update_1998/1998_ 12.pdf. Accessed September 14, 2015.
35. Sarrafian SK. Anatomy of the foot and ankle: descriptive, topographic, functional. 2nd edition. Philadelphia: JP Lippincott Company; 1993. p. 58–65.
36. Zwipp H. Chirurgie des Fusses. Wien, New York: Springer Verlag; 1994. p. 17–9.
37. Williams PL. Gray's anatomy. 38th edition. Edinburgh; London; New York; Philadelphia; Sydney (Australia): Churchill Livingstone; Toronto; 1995. p. 886.
38. Ballal MS, Walker CR, Molloy AP. The anatomical footprint of the Achilles tendon: a cadaveric study. Bone Joint J 2014;96B(10):1344–8.
39. Lohrer H, Arentz S, Nauck T, et al. The Achilles tendon insertion is crescent-shaped: an in vitro anatomic investigation. Clin Orthop Relat Res 2008;466: 2230–7.
40. Maffulli N, Sharma P, Luscombe KL. Achilles tendinopathy: aetiology and management. J R Soc Med 2004;97(10):472–6.
41. Thordarson BD. Foot & ankle. 2nd edition. Lippincott Williams & Wilkins; 2013.
42. Rufai A, Ralphs JR, Benjamin M. Structure and histopathology of the insertional region of the human Achilles tendon. J Orthop Res 1995;13:585–93.
43. Benjamin M, Rufai A, Ralphs JR. The mechanism of formation of bony spurs (enthesophytes) in the Achilles tendon. Arthritis Rheum 2000;43:576–83.
44. Lagergren C, Lindholm A. Vascular distribution on the Achilles tendon - an angiographic and microangiographic study. Acta Chir Scand 1958;776:491–5.
45. Astrom M, Westlin NR. Blood flow in chronic Achilles tendinopathy. Clin Orthop Relat Res 1994;308:166–72.
46. Kirkendall DT, Garrett WE. Function and biomechanics of tendons. Scand J Med Sports 1997;7:62–6.
47. Komi PV, Fukashiro S, Jarvinen M. Biomechanical loading of Achilles tendon during normal locomotion. Clin Sports Med 1992;11:521–31.
48. Canoso JJ, Liu N, Traill MR, et al. Physiology of the retrocalcaneal bursa. Ann Rheum Dis 1988;47(11):910–2.
49. Ruch JA. Haglund's disease. J Am Podiatry Assoc 1974;64(12):1000.

50. Fiamengo SA, Warren RF, Marshall JL. Posterior heel pain associated with a calcaneal step and Achilles tendon calcification. Clin Orthop 1982;167:203–11.

51. Lu CC, Cheng YM, Fu YC, et al. Angle analysis of Haglund syndrome and its relationship with osseous variations and Achilles tendon calcification. Foot Ankle Int 2007;28(2):181–5.

52. James SL, Bates BT, Osternig LR. Injuries to runners. Am J Sports Med 1978; 6(2):40–50.

53. Root ML, Orien WP, Weed JH. Normal and abnormal function of the foot. Clinical Biomechanics, vol. II. Los Angeles (CA): Clin Biomech Corporation; 1977.

54. Sgarlato TE. A compendium of podiatric biomechanics. San Francisco (CA): California College of Podiatric Medicine; 1971. p. 265–81.

55. Sgarlato TE, Morgan J, Shane HS, et al. Tendo achillis lengthening and its effect on foot disorders. J Am Podiatry Assoc 1975;65(9):849–71.

56. Pavlov H, Heneghan MA, Hersh A, et al. The Haglund syndrome: initial and differential diagnosis. Radiology 1982;144(1):83–8.

57. Chauveaux D, Liet P, Le Huec JC, et al. A new radiologic measurement for the diagnosis of Haglund's deformity. Surg Radiol Anat 1991;13(1):39–44.

58. Steffensen JC, Evensen A. Bursitis retrocalcanea achilli. Acta Orthop Scand 1958;27(3):229–36.

59. Kang S, Thordarson D, Charlton T. Insertional Achilles tendinitis and Haglund's deformity. Foot Ankle Int 2012;33(6):487–91.

60. Fuguloang F, Torup D. Bursitis retrocalcanearis. Acta Orthop Scand 1961;30: 315–23.

61. Vega MR, Cavolo DJ, Green RNI, et al. Haglund's deformity. J Am Podiatry Assoc 1984;74(3):129–35.

62. Black AS, Kanat IO. A review of soft tissue calcifications. J Foot Surg 1985;24: 243–50.

63. Maffulli N, Denaro V, Loppini M. Letters to the editor. Foot Ankle Int 2012;33(9): 807–8.

64. Maffulli N, Del Buono A, Testa V, et al. Safety and outcome of surgical debridement of insertional Achilles tendinopathy using a transverse (Cincinnati) incision. J Bone Joint Surg Br 2011;93B:1503–7.

65. Pauker M, Katz K, Yosipovitch Z. Calcaneal ostectomy for Haglund disease. J Foot Surg 1992;31:588–9.

66. Hanft JR, Chang T, Levy AI, et al. Grand rounds: Haglund's deformity and retrocalcaneal, intratendinous spurring. J Foot Ankle Surg 1996;35:362–8.

67. Paavola M, Orava S, Leppilahti J, et al. Chronic Achilles tendon overuse injury: complications after surgical management. An analysis of 432 consecutive patients. Am J Sports Med 2000;28:77–82.

68. Angermann P. Chronic retrocalcaneal bursitis treated by resection of the calcaneus. Foot Ankle 1990;10:285–7.

69. Schepsis AA, Wagner C, Leach RE. Surgical management of Achilles tendon overuse injuries. A long-term follow-up study. Am J Sports Med 1994;22(5): 611–9.

70. Schnieder W, Niehus W, Knahr K. Haglund's syndrome: disappointing results following surgery: a clinical and radiographic analysis. Foot Ankle Int 2000; 21(1):26–30.

71. Huber HM, Waldis M. Die Haglund-Exostoseeine Operationsindikation und ein kleiner Eingriff?. [Haglund's Exostosis—a surgical indication and a minor intervention?] Z Orthop 1989;127:286–90 [in German].

72. Periman MD. Enlargement of the entire posterior aspect of the calcaneus: treatment with the Keck and Kelly calcaneal osteotomy. J Foot Surg 1992;31:424–33.

73. Nesse E, Finsen V. Poor results after resection for Haglund's heel. Analysis of 35 heels treated by arthroscopic removal of bony spurs. Acta Orthop Scand 1994; 65(1):107–9.

74. Kolodziej P, Glisson RR, Nunley JA. Risk of avulsion of the Achilles tendon after partial excision for treatment of insertional tendonitis and Haglund's deformity: a biomechanical study. Foot Ankle Int 1999;20(7):433–7.

75. Nunley JA, Ruskin G, Horst F. Long-term clinical outcomes following the central incision technique for insertional Achilles tendinopathy. Foot Ankle Int 2011;32: 850–5.

76. Maffulli N, Testa V, Capasso G, et al. Calcific insertional Achilles tendinopathy reattachment with bone anchors. Am J Sports Med 2004;32:174–82.

77. Witt BL, Hyer CF. Achilles tendon reattachment after surgical treatment of insertional tendinosis using the suture bridge technique: a case series. J Foot Ankle Surg 2012;51:487–93.

78. Wagner E, Gould J, Bilen E, et al. Change in plantarflexion strength after complete detachment and reconstruction of the Achilles tendon. Foot Ankle Int 2004; 25:800–4.

79. Greenhagen RM, Shinabarger AB, Pearson KT, et al. Intermediate and long-term outcomes of the suture bridge technique for the management of insertional Achilles tendinopathy. Foot Ankle Spec 2013;6:185–90.

80. Pilson H, Brown P, Stitzel J, et al. Single-row versus double-row repair of the distal Achilles tendon: a biomechanical comparison. J Foot Ankle Surg 2012; 51:762–6.

81. Calder JDF, Saxby TS. Surgical treatment of insertional Achilles tendinosis. Foot Ankle Int 2003;24(2):119–21.

82. Johnson KW, Zalavras C, Thordarson DB. Surgical management of insertional calcific Achilles tendinosis with a central tendon splitting approach. Foot Ankle Int 2006;27(4):245–50.

83. Rigby RB, Cottom JM, Vora A. Early weightbearing using Achilles suture bridge technique for insertional Achilles tendinosis: a review of 43 patients. J Foot Ankle Surg 2013;52(5):575–9.

84. Brunner J, Anderson J, O'Malley M, et al. Physician and patient based outcomes following surgical resection of Haglund's deformity. Acta Orthop Belg 2005; 71(6):718–23.

85. Hunt KJ, Cohen BE, Davis WH, et al. Surgical treatment of insertional Achilles tendinopathy with or without flexor hallucis longus tendon transfer: a prospective, randomized study. Foot Ankle Int 2015;36(9):998–1005.

86. Wagner E, Gould JS, Kneidel M, et al. Technique and results of Achilles tendon detachment and reconstruction for insertional Achilles tendinosis. Foot Ankle Int 2006;27:677–84.

87. Carmont MR, Fawdington RA, Mei-Dan O. Endoscopic debridement of the Achilles insertion, bursa, and the calcaneal tubercle with an accessory postero-lateral portal: technique tip. Foot Ankle Int 2011;32:648–50.

88. van Dijk CN, van Dyk CE, Scholten PE, et al. Endoscopic calcaneoplasty. Am J Sports Med 2001;29:185–9.

89. Jerosch J, Schunk J, Sokkar SH. Endoscopic calcaneoplasty (ECP) as a surgical treatment of Haglund's syndrome. Knee Surg Sports Traumatol Arthrosc 2007;15:927–34.

90. Jerosch J. Endoscopic calcaneoplasty. Foot Ankle Clin 2015;20(1):149–65.

91. Ortmann FW, McBryde AM. Endoscopic bony and soft-tissue decompression of the retrocalcaneal space for the treatment of Haglund's deformity and retrocalcaneal bursitis. Foot Ankle Int 2007;28(2):149–53.

92. Wiegerinck JI, Kerkhoffs GM, van Sterkenburg MN, et al. Treatment for insertional Achilles tendinopathy: a systematic review. Knee Surg Sports Traumatol Arthrosc 2013;21(6):1345–55.

93. Bohu Y, Lefèvre N, Bauer T, et al. Surgical treatment of Achilles tendinopathies in athletes. Multicenter retrospective series of open surgery and endoscopic techniques. Orthop Traumatol Surg Res 2009;95(Suppl 1):S72–7.

94. Keck SW, Kelly PJ. Bursitis of the posterior part of the heel; evaluation of the surgical treatment of 18 patients. J Bone Joint Surg Am 1965;47:267–73.

95. Leitze Z, Sella EJ, Aversa JM. Endoscopic decompression of the retrocalcaneal space. J Bone Joint Surg Am 2003;85A(8):1488–96.

96. Berlet G, Smith B, Giza E. Arthroscopic retrocalcaneal burssectomy. In: Philbin T, editor. Surgical techniques in orthopaedics: Achilles tendon disorders. Special edition DVD. Rosemont (IL): American Academy of Orthopaedic Surgeons; 2008.

97. Maquirriain J. Endoscopic Achilles tenodesis: a surgical alternative for chronic insertional tendinopathy. Knee Surg Sports Traumatol Arthrosc 2007;15:940–3.

98. Zadek I. An operation for the cure of achillobursitis. Am J Surg 1939;43(2):542–6.

99. Keck SW, Kelly PJ. Bursitis of the posterior part of the heel: evaluation of surgical treatment of 18 patients. J Bone Joint Surg 1965;47A:267–73.

100. Miller AE, Vogel TA. Haglund's deformity and Keck and Kelly osteotomy, a retrospective analysis. J Foot Surg 1989;28:23–9.

101. Martin D. The Podiatry Institute. The posterior calcaneal osteotomy for retrocalcaneal spur syndromes: a five-year retrospective analysis. Available at: www.podiatryinstitute.com/pdfs/Update_1998/1998_13.pdf. Accessed September 14, 2015.

102. Martin D. Posterior calcaneal osteotomy: a surgical alternative for chronic retrocalcaneal pain. In: Camasta CA, Vickers NS, Reds CS, editors. Reconstructive surgery of the foot and leg update 95. Tucker (GA): Podiatry Institute Publishing; 1995. p. 13–8.

103. Vernois J, Redfern D, Ferraz L, et al. Minimally Invasive surgery osteotomy of the hindfoot clinics in podiatric medicine and surgery. Clin Podiatr Med Surg 2015; 32(3):419–34.

Endoscopic Ankle Lateral Ligament Graft Anatomic Reconstruction

Frederick Michels, MD[a],*, Guillaume Cordier, MD[b],
Stéphane Guillo, MD[b], Filip Stockmans, MD, PhD[c,d],
ESKKA-AFAS Ankle Instability Group

KEYWORDS

- Ankle instability • Anterior talofibular ligament • Calcaneofibular ligament
- Endoscopic reconstruction • Tendoscopy • Gracilis tendon • Autograft • Allograft

KEY POINTS

- Chronic ankle instability is a common complication after an ankle sprain.
- Recently, there has been a move towards endoscopic treatment of lateral ligament instability.
- The endoscopic approach offers the possibility of assessing and addressing associated intra-articular lesions.
- A good knowledge of the local anatomy is indispensable; the anterior tibiofibular ligament, the lateral gutter, the peroneal tendons, and the subtalar joint are used as anatomic landmarks for endoscopic orientation.
- The technique is technically demanding and cadaveric training is needed. If the surgeon lacks the necessary technical skills and experience in endoscopic ankle surgery, open reconstruction is recommended.

INTRODUCTION

Ankle sprains are the most common injuries sustained during sports activities. The most commonly injured ligaments of the ankle are the anterior talofibular ligament (ATFL) and the calcaneofibular ligament (CFL). Most ankle sprains recover fully with

Disclosure Statement: The Biomet Sports Medicine Department paid for a part of the drawings seen in this article.
[a] Orthopaedic Department, AZ Groeninge Kortrijk, Burg Vercruysselaan 5, Kortrijk 8500, Belgium; [b] Orthopaedic Department, Mérignac Sport Clinic, 2 Rue Georges Negrevergne, Mérignac 33700, France; [c] Orthopaedic Department, AZ Groeninge Kortrijk, Loofstraat 43, Kortrijk 8500, Belgium; [d] Department of Development and Regeneration, Faculty of Medicine, University of Leuven Campus Kortrijk, Etienne Sabbelaan 53, Kortrijk 8500, Belgium
* Corresponding author.
E-mail address: frederick_michels@hotmail.com

nonsurgical treatment, but up to 20% of patients develop chronic ankle instability.[1–4] If conservative treatment fails, surgical treatment should be considered. The surgical techniques can be divided into anatomic repair, nonanatomic reconstruction, and anatomic reconstruction.

Anatomic repairs are still considered the gold standard for treatment of symptomatic chronic instability.[5–8] The Broström procedure is a true repair of the lateral ligaments and is often associated with the Gould procedure, which uses the extensor retinaculum to augment the repair.[9,10]

Recently, there has been a move towards endoscopically assisted or full endoscopic repair of the lateral ligaments.[4,5,7,11–13] The endoscopic approach offers the possibility of assessing and addressing associated intra-articular lesions.[14–16]

Nonanatomic procedures have fallen out of favor, because they can overconstrain the talocrural and subtalar joints, resulting in limited range of motion and the long-term development of degenerative arthritis.[8,17,18]

However, an anatomic repair is not always the best option. Several contraindications to anatomic repair have been described in **Box 1**.[5,6,8,14,19,20] A reconstruction should be considered in these cases.

Several studies have published good results using a hamstring autograft or allograft to perform the reconstruction.[2,3,21–24] The peroneal tendons should no longer be used as a graft, as they are important dynamic stabilizers of the hindfoot.[21,25]

This article describes an endoscopic technique, using a step-by-step approach to reconstruct the ATFL and CFL with a gracilis graft.[18,26–28]

SURGICAL TECHNIQUE
Preoperative Planning

The primary indication for operative intervention is the failure of nonsurgical management. Physical examination is essential to confirm the diagnosis of ankle instability. The anterior drawer test and talar tilt test should be performed, and any varus malalignment should be noted.

Plain standing radiographs should be obtained. A comparative Saltzman view (or Méary view) is useful to assess hindfoot alignment. In case of a hindfoot varus, a calcaneal osteotomy should be considered. If a calcaneal osteotomy is associated with a ligament reconstruction, the osteotomy should be performed before the ligament reconstruction to avoid damage to the calcaneal tunnel. Stress radiographs may be helpful, but there are still some concerns as to their the accuracy.

MRI scan can be useful in diagnosing associated injuries. MRI has high specificity and positive predictive value in diagnosing lesions of the ATFL, CFL, and osteochondral lesions; however, its sensitivity is low.[29,30]

Box 1
Indications for reconstruction

- Failed anatomic repair
- High body mass index
- Incompetent ATFL, as seen during arthroscopic examination
- Congenital ligament hyperlaxity
- Heavy labor occupation or sports requirements
- An ossicle with size ≥ 1 cm

Patient Preparation and Positioning

The patient is positioned on his or her side, with a support under the lower leg that allows the ankle to be positioned either laterally or vertically by rotating the leg. This set-up makes it possible to perform anterior and lateral ankle arthroscopy during the same procedure. A tourniquet is applied proximally on the thigh and set to between 250 and 300 mm Hg.

The following landmarks are externally marked: the lateral malleolus, the anterior joint line, the tibialis anterior tendon, the base of the fifth metatarsal, and the peroneal tendons (**Fig. 1**).

A 4 mm 30° arthroscope and a 4.5 full radius synovial shaver are used. No distraction is used.

Surgical Approach

Four arthroscopic portals are used (**Fig. 2**, **Table 1**). Portal 1 (P1) is the anterior medial portal, located medially to the tibialis anterior tendon at the level of the anterior joint line. Portal 2 (P2) is the anterior lateral portal, located anterolaterally almost 1 cm below the joint line, just above the talar insertion of the ATFL. Portal 3 (P3) is positioned at the sinus tarsi, at the level of the superior side of the peroneus brevis and at the posterior side of the extensor retinaculum. Portal 4 (P4), the retromalleolar portal, is optional.

The portals should be created using the nick and spread technique to avoid injury to the superficial neurovascular structures.

Preparation of the Gracilis Graft

The gracilis is folded around a ToggleLoc (Biomet, Warsaw, Indiana) (**Fig. 3**). The central point is sutured together over a length of 10 mm, in preparation for entry into the fibular tunnel. It is important that the wires of the ToggleLoc can move freely. The end used to reconstruct the ATFL measures 30 mm, of which 15 mm are used to create the reconstructed ATFL; 15 mm are used for fixation in the talar tunnel. The end used to reconstruct the CFL is folded to obtain a final length of approximately 55 mm, of which 20 to 25 mm are used to create the new CFL; the remainder is used for fixation in the calcaneal tunnel.

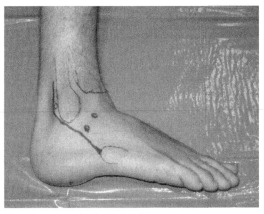

Fig. 1. External landmarks are marked on the skin.

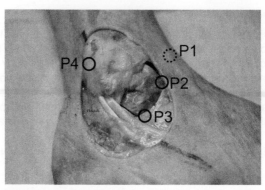

Fig. 2. Endoscopic portals.

Step 1: Anterior Ankle Arthroscopy

First, the ankle is positioned in dorsal decubitus. The skin is incised using the tip of a number 15 scalpel blade, with subsequent blunt dissection using a hemostat spreading technique. A scope is introduced through the standard anteromedial portal (P1). Subsequently, an anterolateral portal is made using the light beam from the scope. First, a needle is used to confirm the intra-articular position and the possible access to the lateral gutter. The joint is then inspected for associated lesions, which are treated if needed.

The shaver is used to debride the synovial tissue covering the anterior tibiofibular ligament (ATiFL). Any scar and inflamed tissue is resected. The ligament is followed to its inferior insertion on the fibula just above the insertion of the ATFL. The soft tissue between the ATiFL and the ATFL is resected. A percutaneously placed needle in the superior part of the ATFL may be useful for orientation and to avoid immediate resection of the ATFL. First the superior part of the ATFL is debrided, followed by the lateral part. Finally, the entire course of both the ATiFL and ATFL is visible (**Fig. 4**). After assessment of the ATFL remnants, the ligament is resected from its malleolar insertion to its talar insertion.

Table 1 Portals		
Portals	**Location**	**Use**
P1 anteromedial portal	At the level of the anterior joint line medially to the tibialis anterior tendon	• Joint inspection • Visualization during lateral joint dissection
P2 anterolateral portal	1 cm below the level of the anterior joint line laterally to the peroneus tertius tendon	• Lateral joint dissection • Drilling of talar tunnel • Fixation in talar tunnel
P3 sinus tarsi portal	Above the peroneus brevis tendon and posteriorly of the extensor retinaculum	• Drilling of fibular tunnel • Drilling of calcaneal tunnel • Graft insertion • Fixation in fibular and calcaneal tunnel
P4 retromalleolar portal (optional)	1 cm posterior and 2 cm proximal to the tip of the lateral malleolus	• Tendoscopy to inspect and treat associated peroneal lesions • Guidance to locate CFL

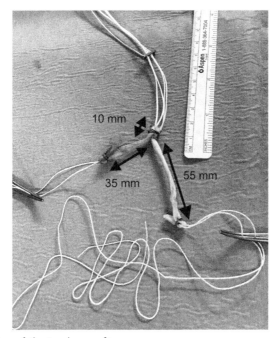

Fig. 3. Preparation of the tendon graft.

Step 2: Lateral Hindfoot Endoscopy

The ankle is placed in lateral decubitus to allow better access around the lateral malleolus. The third portal is created just above the superior border of the peroneus brevis tendon and posteriorly from the extensor retinaculum. With the shaver in portal 3 and

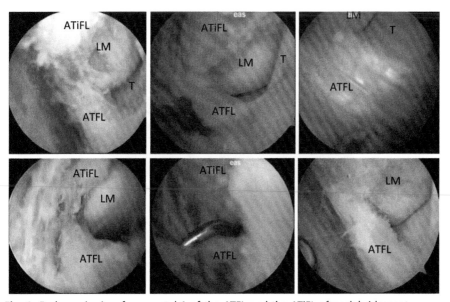

Fig. 4. Endoscopic view from portal 1 of the ATFL and the ATiFL after debridement.

the arthroscope in portal 2, the malleolar attachment of the ATFL and the CFL is prepared. As the insertion sites of the ATFL and CFL on the fibula are confluent, only 1 common tunnel for fixation in the fibula is created.[31] Using portal 3, a guidepin is drilled from the confluent insertion of both ligaments in a posterior and superior direction to reach the posterior cortex of the fibula 3 to 5 cm proximal to the distal tip. The guidepin is overdrilled with a 4.5 diameter drill. Using the same guidepin, the first 10 to 15 mm are over-drilled with a diameter 6 mm (**Fig. 5**). A suture is placed through the eyelet of a Beath pin, which pulls the suture through the tunnel. The suture will be used as a guide wire to pull the graft into the correct position in a subsequent step.

The lateral dissection is continued from anteriorly to posteriorly. Using the subtalar joint and the peroneal tendons as landmarks, the medial part of the tendon sheath is resected. Finally, the insertion of the CFL on the calcaneus is visible behind the peroneal tendons (**Fig. 6**). The lateral border of the subtalar joint is useful for orientation (**Fig. 7**). Alternatively, the retromalleolar portal can be used to dissect the CFL (see optional step).

With the scope still in portal 2, and using portal 3 as a working portal, first a guide pin is drilled; then a tunnel with a diameter of 6 mm is over-drilled towards the medial posterior part of the calcaneus until it perforates the second cortical wall (**Fig. 8**). The Beath pin is used to place a guide wire.

Step 3: Talar Tunnel

With the scope in portal 3, the insertion of the ATFL on the talus is visualized. The insertion site is situated just below the triangular region of the talus, immediately anterior to the joint surface occupied by the lateral malleolus (**Fig. 9**).[31–34] Using a guide pin, a tunnel with a diameter of 5 mm and depth of 20 mm is drilled towards the most posterior part of the medial malleolus (**Figs. 10** and **11**). A blind-ended tunnel directed to the posterior point is the safest option.[35] However, no perforation is allowed, in order to avoid damage to the posteromedial neurovascular bundle. Alternatively, if a transosseous tunnel is preferred, the tunnel should be directed to the most distal part of the medial malleolus (see **Fig. 11**). In this case, a Beath pin is used to pull 1 end of a suture through the tunnel. The suture can be used to pull the end of the graft into the tunnel.

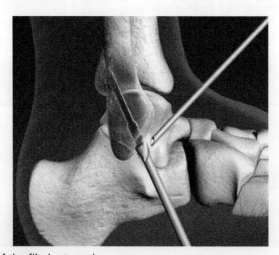

Fig. 5. Drilling of the fibular tunnel.

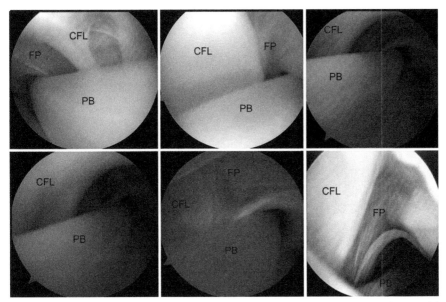

Fig. 6. Visualization of insertion of CFL behind the peroneal tendons (PT) on the calcaneus (C).

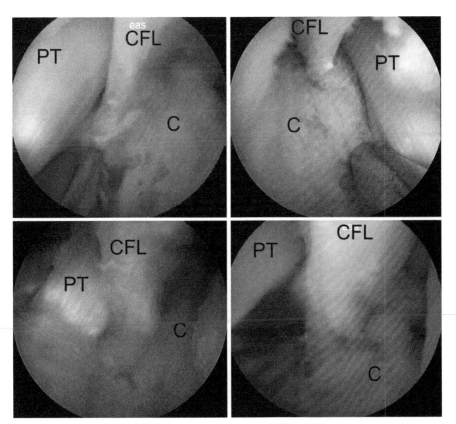

Fig. 7. Endoscopic view of CFL using the subtalar joint (ST) as a landmark.

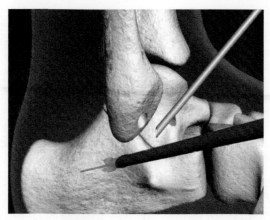

Fig. 8. Drilling of the calcaneal tunnel.

Step 4: Graft Fixation

Using portal 3, the ToggleLoc is pulled inside the fibular tunnel. With this device, working as a pulley, the central part of the graft is pulled 5 mm into the fibular tunnel. It is important that the ToggleLoc is in the correct position. The ToggleLoc should stick to the posterior cortex of the fibula and should be orientated longitudinally (**Fig. 12**).

The anterior part is pulled into the talar tunnel with the screw inserter. This is then fixed with a BioCompositeTenodesis Screw (Arthrex, Naples, Florida), with a diameter of 4.75 mm and a length of 15 mm. The ToggleLoc allows the new ATFL to be tightened by an additional 5 mm, if necessary. The other end is pulled through the calcaneus and fixed with a BioCompositeTenodesis Screw, with a diameter of 7 mm and a length of 23 mm. Because of the weaker bone in the calcaneus, slight oversizing of the screw is possible. All fixation is performed by manual tension. During the fixation, the ankle joint is held in a valgus position. Finally, a good fixation of the new ligaments in an anatomic position is obtained (**Fig. 13**). All the portals are closed using absorbable Monocryl 3.0, and a short leg splint is applied.

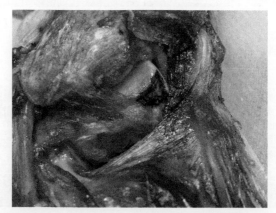

Fig. 9. Insertion of the ATFL just below the triangular region of the talus.

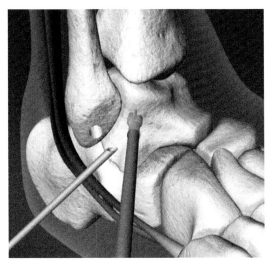

Fig. 10. Drilling of the talar tunnel.

Optional Step: Tendoscopy

After drilling of the fibular tunnel, the retromalleolar portal can be used for dissection of the CFL. The reconstruction can also be performed without using this portal, although it offers some advantages.[36] Tendoscopy is very helpful for assessing and treating associated lesions of the peroneal tendons, such as longitudinal tears, tendon dislocation, and synovitis. It is also very helpful for localizing the insertion site of the CFL.[25]

Portal 4, the retromalleolar portal, is created 1 cm posterior and 2 cm proximal to the tip of the lateral malleolus. The peroneal tendon sheath is incised, and the scope is introduced. The scope is placed anteriorly to the peroneus brevis tendon and carefully

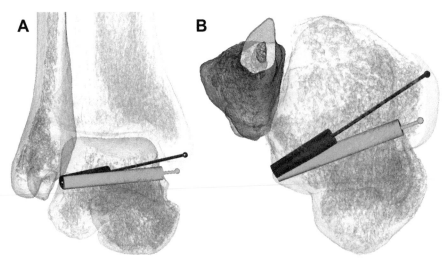

Fig. 11. Bone tunnels. Blind-ended tunnel towards the most posterior point of the medial malleolus (*blue*), transosseous tunnel towards most distal point (*green*). (*A*) Coronal view. (*B*) Axial view.

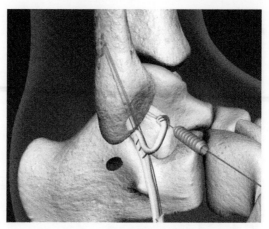

Fig. 12. Fixation in the talar tunnel.

pushed up, distally. The septum of the 2 separated tendon sheaths is visualized at the distal part of the common tunnel. The CFL is visualized more proximally (**Fig. 14**). During tendoscopy, associated lesions of the peroneal tendons are inspected and treated. Using portal 3 as a working portal, a mosquito clamp is used to gain access to the tendon sheath. The view from portal 4 facilitates the resection of the medial part of the common tendon sheath and the underlying fat pad between the septum and the CFL. This creates a working space anterior to the CFL, with the CFL, peroneal tendons, and subtalar joint acting as anatomic landmarks.

Complications and Management

Technical errors

As there are many steps, technical errors are possible. The use of a systematic step-by-step approach should be helpful in avoiding these complications. In case of any doubt, conversion to an open procedure can always be considered (**Table 2**).

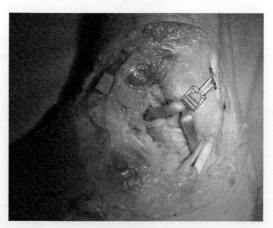

Fig. 13. Final result.

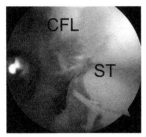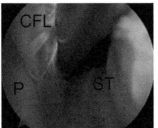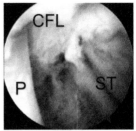

Fig. 14. Tendoscopic view of CFL, peroneus brevis tendon (PB), and fat pad (FP).

Neurologic Lesions

Two recently published cadaveric studies revealed no nerve lesions.[28,37] An anatomic safe zone without important nerve structures was defined as the area surrounded by the superior part of the peroneal tendons, the CFL, the anterior inferior part of the lateral malleolus, and the inferior part of portal 2 (**Fig 18**).[28]

Postoperative Care

The rehabilitation protocol is based on the study published by Pearce.[38] A short period (10–14 days) of immobilization with a short leg splint and elevation of the leg is used to accelerate wound healing and decrease swelling.

Following this, weight bearing is allowed in a walker boot. Patients may remove the boot to mobilize the ankle in the dorsi/plantar flexion range and in inversion/eversion under safe conditions (restricted range of motion of 10°–15° associated with lateral semirigid supports), but they should not walk without protection until week 6.

The early rehabilitation phase occurs between weeks 6 and 10 after surgery. The patient is allowed to walk without bracing. The goals of this phase include increasing strength and range of motion of the entire lower extremity, restoring full ankle/foot active range of motion, and improving gait symmetry to allow for pain-free completion of activities of daily living.

During the late rehabilitation phase (between weeks 8 and 12 after surgery), functional exercises are gradually increased to allow the return to sport between 12 weeks and 4 months following surgery.

Outcomes

The presented step-by-step reconstruction was studied on 14 lower limbs from 7 fresh-frozen cadavers.[28] In all reconstructions, a good stability was obtained. The measurements revealed a good positioning of the reconstructed ligament insertions with a maximal error of 2 mm in most specimens. Anatomic dissection revealed no damage to the surrounding anatomic structures that were at risk.

The benefits of an arthroscopic approach over an open approach have already been shown in other ankle conditions.[18] Studies have shown that converting to an arthroscopic technique can be demanding, with a long learning curve and an increase in surgical time; however, the advantages of preserving the soft-tissue envelope and the improved visualization outweigh these issues. One can see an improved recovery, less pain, a lower rate of soft tissue complications, and improved healing through better preservation of the blood supply.[39]

Clinical studies are being performed and confirm the benefits of these techniques.[18] A database comparing all surgical techniques used to treat ankle instability is recommended as a future goal.

Table 2
Steps and pitfalls

Step	Pitfall	Management
Graft preparation	A graft with too long ends on the fibular of talar site cannot be tensioned sufficiently	Correct graft preparation is mandatory (see **Fig. 2**)
Anterior ankle arthroscopy	Inadequate clearance and dissection increases the risk of technical errors	Sufficient dissection and debridement are necessary
Fibular tunnel	Poor placement of portal 3 can result in misdirection of the fibular tunnel	The exact placement of portal 3 should be determined by the guided tunnel position; a percutaneous needle can be used as a guide
Fibular tunnel	Poor preparation of the tunnel insertion site can result in a fracture of the lateral tunnel wall	Good visualization and sufficient preparation is needed before insertion of the guide pin; the shaver can be used to indicate the correct position
Tendoscopy	The arthroscope can easily pass alongside the tendon sheath	Careful incision of the tendon sheath is needed; small retractors may be helpful when introducing the scope under direct visualization
Talar tunnel	The correct insertion of the ATFL is on the border of the sinus tarsi; when drilling, the guide pin may glide into the sinus tarsi, which can cause incorrect placement of the talar tunnel	A good knowledge of the correct insertion site is indispensable; a tunnel directed to the posterior border of the medial malleolus allows a more perpendicular orientation of the drill bit to the bone surface and avoids gliding
Talar tunnel	A tunnel towards the posterior border of the medial malleolus can damage the neurovascular bundle	A blind tunnel with a maximal depth of 20 mm should be used; if a transosseous tunnel is desired, the tunnel should be directed to the tip of the medial malleolus
Calcaneal tunnel	The correct insertion of the CFL is behind the peroneal tendons	It is necessary to push the peroneal tendons distally to avoid damage to the tendons and allow good tunnel placement
Graft in fibular tunnel	Correct placement of the ToggleLoc is important; if the ToggleLoc is placed behind the peroneal tendon(s), the fixation will be instable (**Fig. 15**); if the ToggleLoc is in a transverse position, the peroneal tendons will be damaged by the sharp edges of the device (**Fig. 16**)	Often the ToggleLoc can be palpated subcutaneously; in case of any doubt, fluoroscopy is recommended
Graft in talar tunnel	It may be difficult to insert the graft end into the talar tunnel	The graft end should not be too bulky; cleaning the entrance of the tunnel with the shaver may be helpful
Graft in calcaneal tunnel	The screw should countersink under the level of the bone surface to avoid protrusion and irritation of the peroneal tendons (**Fig. 17**)	Good visualization during and after screw insertion is needed. The peroneal tendons should be pushed aside to allow this; a coloured screw can be checked more easily than a translucent screw

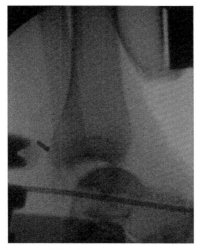

Fig. 15. ToggleLoc behind peroneal tendons.

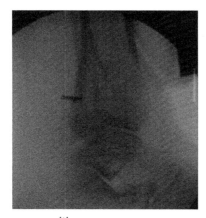

Fig. 16. ToggleLoc in transverse position.

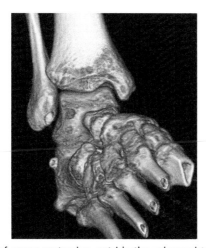

Fig. 17. CT-scan image of screw protrusion outside the calcaneal tunnel.

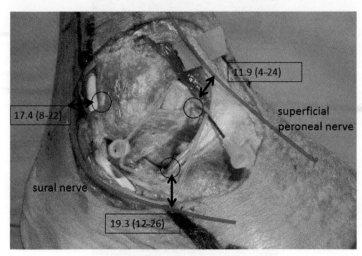

Fig. 18. Safe zone (*green*) and distances to nerves.

SUMMARY

Chronic instability is a common complication of lateral ankle sprains. If nonoperative treatment fails, a surgical repair or reconstruction may be indicated.

Today, endoscopic techniques to treat ankle instability are becoming more popular.

This article described an endoscopic technique, using a step-by-step approach, to reconstruct the ATFL and CFL with a gracilis graft.

Using 4 portals, an endoscopic dissection is performed of the lateral part of the ankle. The insertion sites of the ATFL and CFL are identified, and the ATiFL, the lateral gutter, the peroneal tendons and the subtalar joint are used as anatomic landmarks for endoscopic orientation.

Tunnels are drilled on the anatomic insertion sites. A gracilis graft is prepared, which is then fixed with interference screws in the talus and calcaneus; a button is used in the fibula.

The endoscopic technique is reproducible and safe with regard to the surrounding anatomic structures. Short and midterm results confirm the benefits of this technique.

ACKNOWLEDGMENTS

The ESKKA-AFAS Ankle Instability Group members are as follows: J. Batista, T. Bauer, J. Calder, W.J. Choi, A. Ghorbani, M. Glazebrook, S. Guillo, J. Karlsson, S.W. Kong, J.W. Lee, P.G. Mangone, F. Michels, A. Molloy, C. Nery, S. Ozeki, C. Pearce, A. Perera, H. Pereira, B. Pijnenburg, F. Raduan, J.W. Stone, M. Takao, Y. Tourné.

REFERENCES

1. Broström L. Sprained ankles. V. Treatment and prognosis in recent ligament ruptures. Acta Chir Scand 1966;132:537–50.

2. Caprio A, Oliva F, Treia F, et al. Reconstruction of the lateral ankle ligaments with allograft in patients with chronic ankle instability. Foot Ankle Clin N Am 2006;11:597–605.

3. Coughlin MJ, Schenck RC, Grebing BR, et al. Comprehensive reconstruction of the lateral ankle for chronic instability using a free gracilis graft. Foot Ankle Int 2004;25:231–41.
4. Giza E, Shin EC, Wong SE, et al. Arthroscopic suture anchor repair of the lateral ligament ankle complex: a cadaveric study. Am J Sports Med 2013;41:2567–72.
5. Acevedo JI, Mangone PG. Arthroscopic lateral ligament reconstruction. Tech Foot Ankle Surg 2011;10:111–6.
6. Clanton TO, Viens NA, Campbell KJ, et al. Anterior talofibular ligament ruptures, part 2. Am J Sports Med 2013;42:412.
7. Corte-Real NM, Moreira RM. Arthroscopic repair of chronic lateral ankle instability. Foot Ankle Int 2009;30:213–7.
8. Guillo S, Bauer T, Lee JW, et al. Consensus in chronic ankle instability: aetiology, assessment, surgical indications and place for arthroscopy. Orthop Traumatol Surg Res 2013;99:411–9.
9. Broström L. Sprained ankles. VI Surgical treatment of "chronic" ligament ruptures. Acta Chir Scand 1966;132:551–65.
10. Gould N, Seligson D, Gassman J. Early and late repair of lateral ligament of the ankle. Foot Ankle 1980;1:84–9.
11. Kim ES, Lee KT, Park JS, et al. Arthroscopic anterior talofibular ligament repair for chronic ankle instability with a suture anchor technique. Orthopedics 2011;34(4). http://dx.doi.org/10.3928/01477447-20120228-03.
12. Nery C, Raduan F, Del Buono A, et al. Arthroscopic-assisted Broström-Gould for chronic ankle instability: a long-term follow-up. Am J Sports Med 2011;39:2381–8.
13. Takao M, Matsui K, Stone JW, et al. Arthroscopic anterior talofibular ligament repair for lateral instability of the ankle. Knee Surg Sports Traumatol Arthrosc 2015. http://dx.doi.org/10.1007/s00167-015-3638-0.
14. Ferkel RD, Chams RN. Chronic lateral instability: arthroscopic findings and long-term results. Foot Ankle Int 2007;28:24–31.
15. Hinterman B, Boss A, Schäfer D. Arthroscopic findings in patients with chronic ankle instability. Am J Sports Med 2002;30:402–9.
16. Komenda GA, Ferkel RD. Arthroscopic findings associated with the unstable ankle. Foot Ankle Int 1999;20:708–13.
17. Bahr R, Pena F, Shine J, et al. Biomechanics of ankle ligament reconstruction. An in vitro comparison of the Broström repair, Watson-Jones reconstruction, and a new anatomic reconstruction technique. Am J Sports Med 1997;25:424–32.
18. Guillo S, Archbold P, Perera A, et al. Arthroscopic anatomic reconstruction of the lateral ligaments of the ankle with gracilis autograft. Arthrosc Tech 2014;22(3):e593–8.
19. Kim BS, Choi WJ, Kim YS, et al. The effect of an ossicle of the lateral malleolus on ligament reconstruction of chronic lateral ankle instability. Foot Ankle Int 2010;31:191–6.
20. Vega J, Golano P, Pellegrino A, et al. All-inside arthroscopic lateral collateral ligament repair for ankle instability with a knotless suture anchor technique. Foot Ankle Int 2013;34:1701–9.
21. Jung HG, Kim TH, Park JY, et al. Anatomic reconstruction of the anterior talofibular and calcaneofibular ligaments using a semitendinosus tendon allograft and interference screws. Knee Surg Sports Traumatol Arthrosc 2012;20:1432–7.
22. Paterson R, Cohen B, Taylor MD, et al. Reconstruction of the lateral ligaments of the ankle using semi-tendinosis graft. Foot Ankle Int 2000;21:413–9.

23. Takao M, Oae K, Uchio Y, et al. Anatomical reconstruction of the lateral ligaments of the ankle with a gracilis autograft: a new technique using an interference fit anchoring system. Am J Sports Med 2005;33:814–23.

24. Wang B, Xu XY. Minimally invasive reconstruction of lateral ligaments of the ankle using semitendinosus autograft. Foot Ankle Int 2013;34:711–5.

25. Ziai P, Benca E, von Skrbensky G, et al. The role of the peroneal tendons in passive stabilisation of the ankle joint: an in vitro study. Knee Surg Sports Traumatol Arthrosc 2013;21:1404–8.

26. Guillo S, Cordier G, Sonnery-Cottet B, et al. Anatomical reconstruction of the anterior talofibular and calcaneofibular ligaments with an all-arthroscopic surgical technique. Orthop Traumatol Surg Res 2014;100:S413–7.

27. Guillo S, Takao M, Karlson J, et al. Ankle Instability Group. Arthroscopic anatomical reconstruction ot the lateral ankle ligaments. Knee Surg Sports Traumatol Arthrosc 2015. http://dx.doi.org/10.1007/s00167-015-3789-z.

28. Michels F, Cordier G, Burssens A, et al. Endoscopic reconstruction of CFL and the ATFL with a gracilis graft: a cadaveric study. Knee Surg Sports Traumatol Arthrosc 2015. http://dx.doi.org/10.1007/s00167-015-3779-1.

29. Joshy S, Abdulkadir U, Chaganti S, et al. Accuracy of MRI scan in the diagnosis of ligamentous and chondral pathology in the ankle. Foot Ankle Surg 2010;16: 78–80.

30. Takao M, Innami K, Matsushita T, et al. Arthroscopic and magnetic resonance image appearance and reconstruction of the anterior talofibular ligament in cases of apparent functional ankle instability. Am J Sports Med 2008;36;1542–7.

31. Neuschwander TB, Indresano AA, Hughes TH, et al. Footprint of the lateral ligament complex of the ankle. Foot Ankle Int 2013;34:582–6.

32. Burks RT, Morgan J. Anatomy of the lateral ankle ligaments. Am J Sports Med 1994;22:72–7.

33. Golanó P, Vega J, de Leeuw PA, et al. Anatomy of the ankle ligaments: a pictorial essay. Knee Surg Sports Traumatol Arthrosc 2010;18:557–69.

34. Taser F, Shafiq Q, Ebraheim NA. Anatomy of lateral ankle ligaments and their relationship to bony landmarks. Surg Radiol Anat 2006;28:391–7.

35. Michels F, Guillo S, Vanrietvelde F, et al. How to drill the talar tunnel in ATFL reconstruction? Knee Surg Sports Traumatol Arthrosc 2016. http://dx.doi.org/10.1007/s00167-015-4018-0.

36. Guillo S, Michels F, Cordier G, et al. Endoscopie latérale de cheville. In: Société Française d'Arthroscopie, editor. L'arthroscopie. Issy-les-Moulineaux cedex: Elsevier Masson SAS; 2015. p. 1293–8.

37. Thès A, Klouche S, Ferrand M, et al. Assessment of the feasibility of arthroscopic visualization of the lateral ligaments of the ankle: a cadaveric study. Knee Surg Sports Traumatol Arthrosc 2015. http://dx.doi.org/10.1007/s00167-015-3804-4.

38. Pearce CJ, Tourné Y, Zellers J, et al. ESKKA-AFAS Ankle Instability Group. Rehabilitation after anatomical ankle ligament repair or reconstruction. Knee Surg Sports Traumatol Arthrosc 2016. http://dx.doi.org/10.1007/s00167-016-4051-z.

39. Matsui K, Takao M, Miyamoto W, et al. Early recovery after arthroscopic repair compared to open repair of the anterior talofibular ligament for lateral instability of the ankle. Arch Orthop Trauma Surg 2016;1:93–100.

Arthroscopic Subtalar, Double, and Triple Fusion

 CrossMark

Richard Walter, FRCS (Tr&Orth), MSc, Stephen Parsons, FRCS (Tr&Orth),
Ian Winson, FRCS (Tr&Orth)*

KEYWORDS

- Arthroscopic • Subtalar • Triple • Arthrodesis • Fusion

KEY POINTS

- An arthroscopic approach to hindfoot arthrodesis minimizes damage to the soft tissue envelope, with the aim of reducing wound complications, inpatient stay, and time to fusion.
- Either 2 or 3 sinus tarsi portals can be used to prepare all 3 joints of the triple complex for fusion.
- Cannulated screws are used for fixation.
- Complex deformity can be corrected through an arthroscopic triple fusion, although severe bone shape abnormality or significant bone loss, for example after calcaneal fracture malunion, typically requires an open approach.

INTRODUCTION: NATURE OF THE PROBLEM

Triple arthrodesis is an established procedure used in the treatment of painful and deforming conditions of the hindfoot, after the failure of nonoperative treatments. Typical indications are posttraumatic arthrosis, primary osteoarthrosis, inflammatory arthritis, tarsal coalition, and fixed planovalgus and cavovarus deformities. The aim is to produce a stiffer but well-aligned hindfoot with significantly less pain. When disease or deformity are limited to the subtalar joint then this can be arthrodesed in isolation, although in the presence of transverse tarsal joint involvement or rotational deformity the talonavicular joint and, if required, the calcaneocuboid joint should be included in the fusion.

Hindfoot fusion procedures have typically been performed through open incisions, with significant reported rates of nonunion, wound complications, and nerve injury.[1–6] In recent years, arthroscopic ankle arthrodesis has become widely accepted, with several studies suggesting benefits compared with open arthrodesis in terms of union time, functional outcome, length of inpatient stay, and blood loss.[7–11] Applying arthroscopic techniques to triple joint arthrodesis might be expected to produce similar

Disclosures: The authors have nothing to disclose.
Department of Trauma and Orthopaedics, Sports and Orthopaedic Clinic, Bristol Spire Hospital, Redland Road, Bristol BS6 6UT, UK
* Corresponding author.
E-mail address: ianwinson@doctors.org.uk

benefits. Several small series of arthroscopic subtalar fusions[5,12–23] and double and triple fusions[24,25] have reported encouraging results. The ability to prepare the 3 joints largely through 2 sinus tarsi portals has been demonstrated in cadavers.[26]

This article describes a technique for performing arthroscopic subtalar, double, and triple fusion through a sinus tarsi approach, and reviews the reported results to date.

INDICATIONS/CONTRAINDICATIONS

Box 1 lists the indications and contraindications. Note that most of the relative contraindications probably apply to open techniques of surgery, with the single exception of severe deformity associated with bone loss.

SURGICAL TECHNIQUE/PROCEDURE
Preoperative Planning

A thorough history and clinical examination together with standing radiographs usually confirm the diagnosis and source of any pain. If doubt exists, for example in cases with multiple arthritic joints, targeted injection of local anesthetic confirms the extent to which a given joint is contributing to the patient's overall pain, and therefore the extent to which arthrodesis of the joint is likely to provide longer-term relief.

A decision must be made regarding whether to perform an isolated subtalar joint arthrodesis, or a double or triple arthrodesis. When the indication for surgery is painful arthritis, all joints that are severely painful are included. When the aim of surgery is to correct deformity, the relationship of the hindfoot to the midfoot is important. The talonavicular and calcaneocuboid joints are arthrodesed if significant rotational deformity

---

Box 1
Indications and contraindications

Indications

- All causes of end-stage hindfoot arthritis
- Symptomatic hindfoot deformity
- In particular, an arthroscopic approach is of use in patients with compromise of the soft tissue envelope; for example:
  - The elderly
  - Inflammatory arthritides
  - Long-term steroid use
  - Posttraumatic arthrosis with previous scars, skin grafts, or flaps

Contraindications (absolute)

- Active infection

Contraindications (relative)

- Severe compromise of the soft tissue envelope
- Significant bone shape deformity or bone loss requiring correction (eg, correction of calcaneal height after fracture malunion)
- Continued smoking
- Neuropathy (eg, the active stage of Charcot neurarthropathy)
- Vascular compromise (severity should be assessed preoperatively)

is present after the subtalar joint position has been corrected. Overall, when possible, the calcaneocuboid joint is left free, to allow it to contribute a little motion to lateral column flexibility for accommodating uneven ground.

Patients are advised to stop smoking before undergoing surgery, because it is a proven risk factor for nonunion after subtalar fusion[27] and for delayed wound healing, infection, and persistent pain after foot surgery.[28] A rheumatology opinion is sought before asking patients to stop anti–tumor necrosis factor medications for the perioperative period, in order to minimize the risk of infection. Although it seems that these drugs are not the cause of increased rates of infection, the consequences of a chance infection can be serious. Doppler studies and a vascular surgery consultation are obtained if the history, examination, or ankle brachial pulse index indicates arterial insufficiency.

Choice of Arthroscopic Approach

Various arthroscopic approaches can be used to prepare the subtalar joint. The most commonly reported approaches in the literature are the posterior approach (posteromedial and posterolateral portals) and the lateral approach (posterolateral and anterolateral portals). The authors favor the 2-portal sinus tarsi approach, because it allows the patient to be placed in a semilateral position, which is considered to be safer than the prone position for posterior-approach arthroscopy; it avoids the posterolateral portal, which has been associated with a significant risk of sural nerve damage[29–32]; and it allows access to all 3 facets of the subtalar joint, the calcaneocuboid joint, and the plantar-lateral two-thirds of the talonavicular joint.[26]

Preparation and Patient Positioning

- General and/or regional anesthesia.
- A World Health Organization checklist modified for the foot and ankle is performed to minimize the risk to patient safety.
- Prophylactic intravenous antibiotics should be administered.
- The patient is placed in a semilateral position with a large sandbag under the ipsilateral buttock, and the limb to be operated is positioned on a foam cushion or similar support with the foot hanging fairly free (**Fig. 1**).
- Joint distraction is not required.
- A thigh tourniquet is inflated (although the procedure can be performed without tourniquet if required).
- The skin is prepared and draped just above the knee to allow intraoperative movement of the limb, and to allow visual assessment of rotational alignment.
- Consideration should be given to how to collect extravasated fluid.

Surgical Approach

- A 2-portal sinus tarsi approach can be used to access all 3 joints of the triple complex.
- Initial inflation is performed with 10 to 15 mL of fluid injected if possible into the sinus tarsi.
- The proximal portal is marked just above the angle of Gissane and the distal portal just above the palpable anterior process of the calcaneum (**Fig. 2**).
- A nick-and-spread" dissection is used to avoid damage to nerve branches when establishing portals.
- A 4.5-mm 30° arthroscope is inserted (**Fig. 3**).

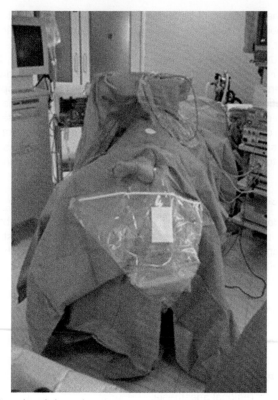

Fig. 1. The positioned and draped patient.

Surgical Procedure

Subtalar joint

Soft tissue resectors (eg, 3.5-mm and 4.8-mm Cuda, CONMED Linvatec, Largo, FL) are used to remove enough soft tissue from the anterolateral aspect of the posterior facet to visualize the joint. A burr (4.5-mm Vortex or Spherical CONMED Linvatec, Largo, FL) is then used to decorticate the posterior facet to expose bleeding cancellous bone, starting anterolaterally and working posteriorly and medially (**Figs. 4** and **5**). The flexor hallucis longus tendon can be visualized, and represents the posterior

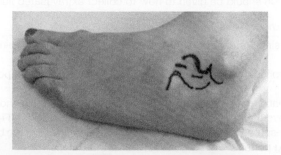

Fig. 2. Landmarks and portals for sinus tarsi approach arthroscopy.

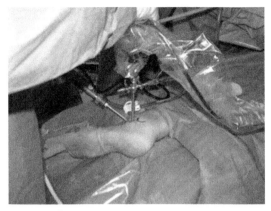

Fig. 3. The 2 sinus tarsi portals in use.

medial limit of the posterior facet. After decortication of the posterior facet, the middle and anterior facets are visualized and sequentially decorticated (**Figs. 6 and 7**). If the intention is to do an isolated subtalar joint fusion, care should be taken not to progress through the anterior facet of the subtalar joint into the talonavicular joint.

Talonavicular joint
Access to the talonavicular joint for decortication is from inferior to superior and from lateral to medial. If required, fluoroscopy with a burr in situ can give information on how far dorsomedially decortication has reached. Typically, in excess of two-thirds of the joint can be prepared from the sinus tarsi portals, although the subchondral plate of the navicular tuberosity is left intact to provide strength for subsequent screw fixation. If further medial decortication is preferred, additional dorsolateral

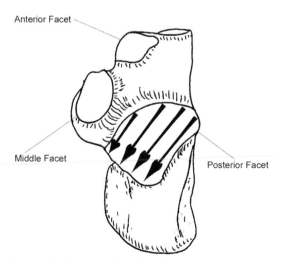

Fig. 4. Direction of posterior facet subtalar decortication.

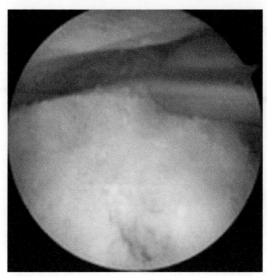

Fig. 5. Burr decortication of the posterior facet of the subtalar joint.

and/or dorsomedial portals can be established, but great care must be taken to avoid neurovascular injury.

Calcaneocuboid joint

If required, this can be prepared through the sinus tarsi portals, working superior to inferior and typically medial to lateral. To gain initial access to the superior part of the joint some burr resection of the overhanging anterior process of the calcaneum is typically required. If required, an additional portal can be placed low on the line of the calcaneocuboid joint.

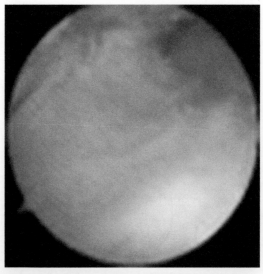

Fig. 6. Junction of the middle and posterior facets of the subtalar joint.

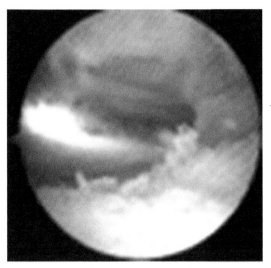

Fig. 7. Decortication of the middle facet of the subtalar joint.

Stabilization

The tourniquet can be released at this stage. An assistant supports the foot with a flat surface in the desired position. Further stab incisions are created to pass cannulated partial-threaded screws. One or wo 6.5-mm or 8-mm screws are used to compress and stabilize the subtalar joint, from the posterior-inferior aspect of the calcaneum to the talar body (**Fig. 8**). One screw (either 4 mm or 6.5 mm depending on skeletal size) from the navicular tuberosity to the talar body is often sufficient to stabilize the talonavicular joint. This screw can be supplemented by a further dorsal screw through the navicular. In addition, a 6.5-mm screw is placed from the posterior aspect of the calcaneum to the centre of the cuboid bone, taking care not to exit the plantar aspect of the bones (or smaller anterolateral to posteromedial cuboid to calcaneum screws can be used; **Figs. 9** and **10**). Fluoroscopic images are checked and saved.

Closure

Wounds are closed with simple sutures. Nonadherent dressings, and a below-knee plaster slab are applied.

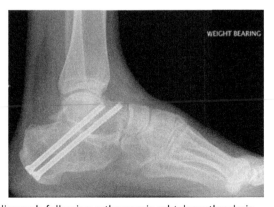

Fig. 8. Lateral radiograph following arthroscopic subtalar arthrodesis.

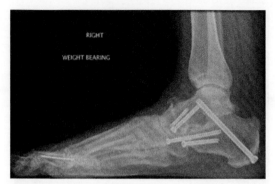

Fig. 9. Lateral radiograph following arthroscopic triple fusion.

Postoperative Care

- Touch weight bearing with crutches in a below-knee plaster slab for 2 weeks.
- See in the outpatient clinic 2 weeks postoperatively to check wounds, remove sutures, and apply a full below-knee cast.
- At 2 weeks postoperatively, begin weight bearing as able in cast (isolated subtalar arthrodesis) or continue touch weight bearing (double or triple arthrodesis).

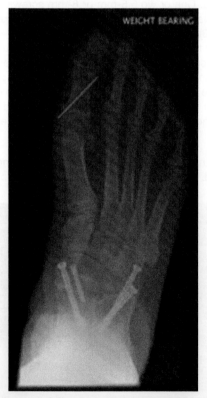

Fig. 10. Dorsoplantar radiograph following arthroscopic triple fusion.

- Weight bear as comfort allows in cast or removable boot from 6 to 8 weeks postoperatively until 12 weeks.
- See in the outpatient clinic 12 weeks postoperatively with standing radiographs on arrival, and leave free of splintage.
- If there is significant doubt about union then continue immobilization for up to 6 months.
- Union is diagnosed in the setting of resolved swelling and symptoms, and absence of lucent lines on radiographs. If a patient has residual symptoms, swelling, or radiographic lucent lines, and does not show clinical or radiographic progress between outpatient appointments, computed tomography can be used to assess the state of union.

COMPLICATIONS AND MANAGEMENT

In general, all of these complications apply to open techniques and the incidence is generally lower than with the open equivalent (**Table 1**).

OUTCOMES

Table 2 summarizes published results of arthroscopic subtalar arthrodesis, and **Table 3** gives published results of arthroscopic triple arthrodesis.

Table 1 Complications and management	
Complication	**Notes**
Thromboembolism	Early mobilization of the limb is a major prophylaxis. When possible we use mechanical rather than chemical thromboprophylaxis, because of the increased risk of wound complications with anticoagulant medications
Nerve injury	The sinus tarsi portal approach minimizes the risk of sural nerve injury.[26] Occasionally, dorsolateral and dorsomedial portals are required to complete talonavicular joint preparation,[24] and a careful nick-and-spread technique must be used to avoid damage to branches of the deep peroneal and superficial peroneal nerves
Nonunion	This is uncommon. Reversible reasons for nonunion, such as cigarette smoking, steroid use, malnutrition, excessive weight bearing, and surgical site infection, should be identified and corrected. Unless the nonunion is mobile and remains accessible arthroscopically, an open approach is often required to repeat the arthrodesis procedure. Bone grafting is typically only required if associated cysts have led to significant bone loss
Infection	Superficial infection is treated with a course of antibiotics guided by wound swab microbiology results. Deep infection is rare; most commonly it requires early removal of metalwork and debridement of the screw tracks urgently with appropriate antibiotics. After the infection settles, new fixation can be reinserted. If it occurs late in the recovery but before full union, limited debridement and washout combined with suppressive antibiotics can be used until radiological evidence of union is convincing, which sometimes requires computed tomography
Irritation from metalwork	Screws can be removed as a day procedure once successful arthrodesis has been achieved

Table 2
Published results of arthroscopic subtalar arthrodesis

Investigators	Portals	n	Union, n (%)	Time to Union (wk)	Infection, n (%)	Nerve Injury, n (%)	Subsequent Removal of Metalwork, n (%)
Walter et al,[33] 2015	Sinus tarsi	77	75 (97)	15.3	1 (1.3)	1 (1.3)	7 (9)
Narita et al,[20] 2012	PL and PM	8	8 (100)	8	0	0	0
Thaunat et al,[23] 2011	PL and PM	14	11 (79)	unknown	0	1 (7)	1 (7)
Albert et al,[13] 2011	PL and PM	10	10 (100)	6.8	0	0	0
Lee et al,[18] 2010	PL and PM	16	15 (94)	16	1 (6)	0	1 (6)
Beimers et al,[15] 2009	PL, PM, and sinus tarsi	3	3 (100)	6	0	0	0
El Shazly et al,[21] 2009	AL × 2 and PM	9	9 (100)	11.44	0	1 (11)	0
Lee et al,[19] 2008	PL × 2 and PM	10	10 (100)	10	0	0	1 (10)
Carro et al,[16] 2007	PL and PM	4	4 (100)	8	0	0	0
Amendola et al,[14] 2007	PL and PM	11	10 (91)	10	0	0	1 (9)
Glanzmann & Sanhueza-Hernandez,[17] 2007	AL and PL	41	41 (100)	11	0	0	10 (24)
Tasto et al,[22] 2000	AL × 2 and PL	25	25 (100)	8.9	0	0	2 (8)
Ahn et al,[12] 2009	AL × 2 and PL	26	25 (96)	10	Unknown	Unknown	1 (4)
Scranton,[5] 1999	AL × 2 and PL	5	5 (100)	26 (not imaged earlier)	0	0	1 (20)
Scranton,[5] 1999	Open lateral (comparison group)	12	11 (92)	26 (not imaged earlier)	0	0	1 (8)

Abbreviations: AL, anteromedial; PL, posterolateral; PM, posteromedial.

Table 3
Published results of arthroscopic triple arthrodesis

Investigators	Portals	n	Union, n (%)	Time to Union (wk)	Infection	Nerve Injury	Subsequent Removal of Metalwork
Jagodzinski et al,[24] 2015	Sinus tarsi × 2 and dorsolateral	4	4 (100)	15	0	0	0
Lui,[25] 2009	Multiple	10	10 (100)	21	0	0	Unknown

SUMMARY

Arthroscopic subtalar, double, and triple joint arthrodesis is technically feasible and carries the potential benefit compared with open surgery of minimizing damage to the soft tissue envelope. As such, it may be associated with improved recovery and union times and decreased complication rates compared with traditional open approaches.

The sinus tarsi portal arthroscopic approach carries the advantages of avoiding the prone position, minimizing the risk of peripheral nerve injury, and affording good access to all 3 joints of the triple complex. In addition, the excellent access to all parts of the hindfoot complex allows correction of deformity through adequate decortication of all articular facets and consequent mobilization of joints, rather than deformity correction through excessive bony resection.

Arthroscopic surgery of this nature is technically challenging. It must be appreciated that there is a learning curve. During this period, it is wise to ensure that intraoperative imaging is available throughout the procedure in order to assist with navigation, and portals can be orientated to facilitate conversion to an open procedure should it be required. In addition, it is expected that, at first, arthroscopic hindfoot operations will take more time than the equivalent open procedures.

REFERENCES

1. Angus PD, Cowell HR. Triple arthrodesis. A critical long-term review. J Bone Joint Surg Br 1986;68(2):260–5.
2. Davies MB, Rosenfeld PF, Stavrou P, et al. A comprehensive review of subtalar arthrodesis. Foot Ankle Int 2007;28(3):295–7.
3. Easley ME, Davis WH, Anderson RB. Intermediate to long-term follow-up of medial-approach dorsal cheilectomy for hallux rigidus. Foot Ankle Int 1999; 20(3):147–52.
4. Mann RA, Beaman DN, Horton GA. Isolated subtalar arthrodesis. Foot Ankle Int 1998;19(8):511–9.
5. Scranton PE. Comparison of open isolated subtalar arthrodesis with autogenous bone graft versus outpatient arthroscopic subtalar arthrodesis using injectable bone morphogenic protein-enhanced graft. Foot Ankle Int 1999;20(3):162–5.
6. Yuan C-S, Tan X-K, Zhou B-H, et al. Differential efficacy of subtalar fusion with three operative approaches. J Orthop Surg Res 2014;9:115.
7. Nielsen KK, Linde F, Jensen NC. The outcome of arthroscopic and open surgery ankle arthrodesis. Foot Ankle Surg 2008;14(3):153–7.
8. O'Brien TS, Hart TS, Shereff MJ, et al. Open versus arthroscopic ankle arthrodesis: a comparative study. Foot Ankle Int 1999;20(6):368–74.

9. Townshend D, Di Silvestro M, Krause F, et al. Arthroscopic versus open ankle arthrodesis: a multicenter comparative case series. J Bone Joint Surg Am 2013;95(2):98–102.

10. Winson IG, Robinson DE, Allen PE. Arthroscopic ankle arthrodesis. J Bone Joint Surg Br 2005;87(3):343–7.

11. Gougoulias NE1, Agathangelidis FG, Parsons SW. Arthroscopic ankle arthrodesis. Foot Ankle Int 2007;28(6):695–706.

12. Ahn JH, Lee SK, Kim KJ, et al. Subtalar arthroscopic procedures for the treatment of subtalar pathologic conditions: 115 consecutive cases. Orthopedics 2009; 32(12):891.

13. Albert A, Deleu P-A, Leemrijse T, et al. Posterior arthroscopic subtalar arthrodesis: ten cases at one-year follow-up. Orthop Traumatol Surg Res 2011;97(4):401–5.

14. Amendola A, Lee K-B, Saltzman CL, et al. Technique and early experience with posterior arthroscopic subtalar arthrodesis. Foot Ankle Int 2007;28(3):298–302.

15. Beimers L, de Leeuw PAJ, van Dijk CN. A 3-portal approach for arthroscopic subtalar arthrodesis. Knee Surg Sports Traumatol Arthrosc 2009;17(7):830–4.

16. Carro LP, Golanó P, Vega J. Arthroscopic subtalar arthrodesis: the posterior approach in the prone position. Arthroscopy 2007;23(4):445.e1–4.

17. Glanzmann MC, Sanhueza-Hernandez R. Arthroscopic subtalar arthrodesis for symptomatic osteoarthritis of the hindfoot: a prospective study of 41 cases. Foot Ankle Int 2007;28(1):2–7.

18. Lee KB, Park CH, Seon JK, et al. Arthroscopic subtalar arthrodesis using a posterior 2-portal approach in the prone position. Arthroscopy 2010;26(2):230–8.

19. Lee K-B, Saltzman CL, Suh J-S, et al. A posterior 3-portal arthroscopic approach for isolated subtalar arthrodesis. Arthroscopy 2008;24(11):1306–10.

20. Narita N, Takao M, Innami K, et al. Minimally invasive subtalar arthrodesis with iliac crest autograft through posterior arthroscopic portals: a technical note. Foot Ankle Int 2012;33(09):803–5.

21. El Shazly O, Nassar W, El Badrawy A. Arthroscopic subtalar fusion for post-traumatic subtalar arthritis. Arthroscopy 2009;25(7):783–7.

22. Tasto JP, Frey C, Laimans P, et al. Arthroscopic ankle arthrodesis. Instr Course Lect 2000;49:259–80.

23. Thaunat M, Bajard X, Boisrenoult P, et al. Computer tomography assessment of the fusion rate after posterior arthroscopic subtalar arthrodesis. Int Orthopaedics 2011;36(5):1005–10.

24. Jagodzinski NA, Parsons AMJ, Parsons SW. Arthroscopic triple and modified double hindfoot arthrodesis. Foot Ankle Surg 2015;21(2):97–102.

25. Lui TH. Arthroscopic triple arthrodesis in patients with Müller Weiss disease. Foot Ankle Surg 2009;15(3):119–22.

26. Hughes A, Gosling O, McKenzie J, et al. Arthroscopic triple fusion joint preparation using two lateral portals: a cadaveric study to evaluate safety and efficacy. Foot Ankle Surg 2014;20(2):135–9.

27. Easley ME, Trnka HJ, Schon LC, et al. Isolated subtalar arthrodesis. J Bone Joint Surg Am 2000;82(5):613–24.

28. Bettin CC, Gower K, McCormick K, et al. Cigarette smoking increases complication rate in forefoot surgery. Foot Ankle Int 2015;36(5):488–93.

29. Frey C, Gasser S, Feder K. Arthroscopy of the subtalar joint. Foot Ankle Int 1994; 15(8):424–8.

30. Lintz F, Guillard C, Colin F, et al. Safety and Efficacy of a two-portal lateral approach to arthroscopic subtalar arthrodesis: a cadaveric study. Arthroscopy 2013;29(7):1217–23.

31. Lui TH, Chan KB, Chan LK. Portal safety and efficacy of anterior subtalar arthroscopy: a cadaveric study. Knee Surg Sports Traumatol Arthrosc 2010;18(2):233–7.
32. Mouilhade F, Oger P, Roussignol X, et al. Risks relating to posterior 2-portal arthroscopic subtalar arthrodesis and articular surfaces abrasion quality achievable with these approaches: a cadaver study. Orthop Traumatol Surg Res 2011; 97(4):396–400.
33. Walter R., Butler M., Parsons S. Arthroscopic subtalar arthrodesis through the two-portal sinus tarsi approach: a series of 77 cases. Presented at the BOFAS annual scientific meeting, Guildford, November 12, 2015.

Index

Note: Page numbers of article titles are in **boldface** type.

Foot Ankle Clin N Am 21 (2016) 695–726
http://dx.doi.org/10.1016/S1083-7515(16)30062-6
1083-7515/16/$ – see front matter

C

Moving?

Make sure your subscription moves with you!

To notify us of your new address, find your **Clinics Account Number** (located on your mailing label above your name), and contact customer service at:

Email: journalscustomerservice-usa@elsevier.com

800-654-2452 (subscribers in the U.S. & Canada)
314-447-8871 (subscribers outside of the U.S. & Canada)

Fax number: 314-447-8029

Elsevier Health Sciences Division
Subscription Customer Service
3251 Riverport Lane
Maryland Heights, MO 63043

*To ensure uninterrupted delivery of your subscription, please notify us at least 4 weeks in advance of move.

Printed and bound by CPI Group (UK) Ltd, Croydon, CR0 4YY

08/05/2025

01864686-0004